The
Low
Glycal
Diet

PAGE STREET
PUBLISHING CO.

First published in 2015 by
Page Street Publishing Co.
27 Congress Street, Suite 103
Salem, MA 01970
www.pagestreetpublishing.com

Distributed by Macmillan, sales in Canada by The Canadian Manda Group.

18   17   16   15   1   2   3   4   5

ISBN-13: 978-1-62414-182-9
ISBN-10: 1-62424-182-X

Library of Congress Control Number: 2015947360

Cover and book design by Page Street Publishing Co.

Printed and bound in the U.S.A.

Page Street is proud to be a member of 1% for the Planet. Members donate one percent of their sales to one or more of the over 1,500 environmental and sustainability charities across the globe who participate in this program.

The
Low
Glycal
Diet

**HOW TO SHED FAT EFFORTLESSLY
WITHOUT BEING HUNGRY OR CUTTING OUT CARBS**

JEFFREY DUNHAM

M.D., Harvard, Ph.D., M.I.T.

With Martha Murphy

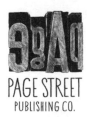

PAGE STREET
PUBLISHING CO.

Contents

FOREWORD

Research overwhelmingly shows that most of us are too fat and that both our bodies and our minds would stay healthier longer if we would get leaner. So, what prevents any of us from taking control of our bodies and getting ourselves leaner and healthier? Quite simply, we lack the knowledge. What knowledge, I hear you ask? Well, several pieces: the knowledge of the signals that tell our body what to do with nutrients, burn them, make muscle or store them as fat; the knowledge of how ingredients in the foods we eat trigger those signals and how that varies throughout the day; the knowledge of how to combine foods so that we can eat with enjoyment, feel satisfied and at the same time get the amount of fat we carry down to a healthy level; lastly and importantly, the knowledge of what specific foods should be combined and how, so that we can stay on a life-long healthy course of eating, and happily so. This book gives you that knowledge and, better yet, gives you instructions and recipes that make it easy to translate that knowledge into good and enjoyable eating.

How do I know this? I know this because I am a physician and psychiatrist whose patients struggle with obesity. They struggle with obesity due to the same factors that make many people obese: diets whose ingredients trigger the body to store too much as fat and that increase the craving for more food than is needed, and misconceptions as to how to eat in a healthy way. Additionally, they struggle with obesity because their mental health conditions make them more vulnerable to overeating. Lastly, they struggle with obesity because the medications that I prescribe to them increase their appetites often markedly. For my patients, learning to stay at a healthy weight and fat percentage is like trying to lift weights on the surface of Jupiter where the gravity is much greater than on the surface of the earth. They have to get very good at learning to eat healthy in order to succeed. I have tried to keep up with how to guide them in this effort and have found the ideas and knowledge in this book, and in its accompanying smart phone app, invaluable in helping my patients.

I also know this because I follow Dr. Dunham's Low-Glycal Diet.™ When I started following the diet, without any other change in my lifestyle or medications, in my mid-50s, I lost 14 pounds of abdominal fat while keeping my lean muscle mass constant. I now easily maintain a healthy 11 percent fat composition by following the diet. Thankfully, this is not difficult. I just follow the plan described in this book. I am not hungry and do not feel deprived of good food.

Lastly, I know this is important not just for me or for my patients but for all of us. The Nurses Health Study demonstrates that the more fat you have, the higher your sugar and insulin levels will be and as a result your long-term health will suffer. I know this from the Kaiser study that shows that increased belly fat in your 40s increases the risk of dementia in your 70s. Excess fat also makes it harder to exercise. The research continues to add to the urgency that we get and keep ourselves at a healthy proportion of fat to muscle.

Dr. Dunham has done the hard work of researching and processing the information that is needed to plan meals in a way that makes this possible. Let him guide you with this book so you can live longer, keep your mind working well, feel good and even enjoy eating!

Joseph Gonzalez-Heydrich, M.D.
Associate Professor of Psychiatry,
Harvard Medical School

INTRODUCTION

This book is about you.

It's about helping you live a leaner, longer and healthier life. When you finish reading it, you'll know what's making you fat (hint: it's not your fault) and what you can do to lose that fat—and keep it off. You'll also understand why being fat "ages" you prematurely—inside and out—and how the food you eat can either speed up that process or slow it down.

There's an old proverb that says, "Give a man a fish and you feed him for a day; teach a man to fish and you feed him for a lifetime." That's why this book starts with a few short chapters about the basic science of how our bodies store fat; by understanding these principles, you'll see *why* The Low-Glycal Diet works, and you'll be more than eager to start the 3-step plan.

I don't want to sell you any packaged meals, programs or supplements. You don't need to shop at expensive organic or health food stores. I want to show you what you can do, right now, to lose fat and extend your healthy years. And you don't need to go any farther than your local supermarket. The meal plans and recipes that are part of the Low-Glycal Diet call for real, delicious, healthful foods.

By the time you've reached the end of this book, you will be able to:

1. Lose fat (not just weight—there's a difference) effortlessly, without being hungry or cutting out carbs

2. Lower your blood pressure, blood sugar and cholesterol levels

3. Lower your risk of diabetes, heart disease, cancer and dementia

4. Have more energy and self-confidence

5. Slow down the aging process

6. Be healthier and live longer

Sound good? It is! That's why I wrote *The Low-Glycal Diet*.

I've been giving this diet (in one form or another) to patients in my medical practice in Palm Springs, California, for the past 12 years. It has evolved from lectures to a diet app for smartphones, and now into this book. I've honed and refined it by recording the body fat of my patients at each visit (using the Bod Pod®, the $25,000 state-of-the-art device used by universities and professional sports teams for measuring body fat) and tracking how their body composition has changed over time. I've seen what works and what doesn't, and have clarified the diet and made it more understandable by answering my patients' questions and responding to thousands of comments from users of the companion app worldwide.

There's so much misinformation out there about diet and nutrition that my patients are understandably confused when they come in for their initial consultation. Even among medical professionals there's no clear consensus, so fad diets fill the void. The correct information *is* out there, however, and is unequivocal, supported by the latest scientific studies published in peer-reviewed, medical journals. The problem is that the average person is unable to make sense of it, and most doctors are unaware of it.

Physicians now seem to get most of their continuing education from pharmaceutical reps who stop by to tout the latest drug. Doctors may read a study or two about a new drug, but after seeing 20 to 30 patients a day, they will rarely have time to read diet studies, which are generally outside the scope of their practices. And because the average length of a patient visit is typically 10 to 15 minutes, there simply isn't enough time to explain the proper diet—even if they knew how. So, when your doctor tells you that you need to lose weight and you ask how, the response will typically be, "Don't eat so much and cut out the fat."

How's that working for you?

The reason doctors give this advice is that about 30 years ago the American Medical Association and the American Heart Association issued guidelines that told us we needed to cut the fat in our diets by 10 percent, from 45 percent of the calories consumed to 35 percent. There wasn't a lot of scientific data to back up this recommendation; it just seemed to make sense at the time. The common belief was that you are what you eat, and if you eat less fat you'll lose fat and lower your risk for heart disease. Well, we all did that, and 30 years later we're eating less fat than we did in 1980, but people are fatter than they ever were. There's an epidemic of obesity in this country, and 10 percent of the adult population has diabetes because of it. We all went on a low-fat diet—and got fatter.

What happened? The food companies took out the fat in processed foods and replaced it with carbohydrates, the most notorious being high-fructose corn syrup. Taking the fat out of food renders it almost tasteless (does anyone really enjoy eating a dry, skinless, boneless chicken breast?), so to make those low-fat and non-fat foods more palatable, they added high-fructose corn syrup (which is sweeter and cheaper than cane sugar). It's almost impossible to find a loaf of bread today without high-fructose corn syrup added. We may be eating less fat but we're eating way more carbohydrates. So is it all those excess carbohydrates that are making us fat? Or is it merely that we're eating more calories? Or, does the answer lie somewhere in between?

I wrote this book to give you a clear, easy-to-understand way to decide what to eat—and when to eat it—to achieve and maintain an ideal weight and slow the aging process. All of the latest research on diet and nutrition supports my advice but, until now, no one has put it all together in a way that's useful for the average person. I'm fighting against billions of dollars in advertising from processed-food manufacturers, who make health claims about their products that are simply wrong, and in my view, almost criminal. This book is my attempt to counter this misinformation overload, and, if enough people read it, a way to curb the current obesity epidemic that threatens to fill the second part of our lives with sickness and disability.

My medical training as a physician-scientist puts me in a unique position to be able to translate advances in medical research into clinical practice. There's a huge gap between the latest research findings and medical practice. It can take 30 or more years for breakthroughs in the lab to filter down to primary care physicians. I want to speed up that process.

Over the past 12 years, I've built a fairly large anti-aging medical practice and have patients from all over the United States and a few foreign countries. My patients include doctors, nurses, business executives and even a few celebrities. I've achieved tremendous success with my patients, but when I look back across those initial years in practice, I wish I'd put more emphasis on what I now consider to be the backbone, the absolutely most essential ingredient of anti-aging medicine. Anti-aging physicians who ignore this will never achieve the truly exceptional outcomes that are possible, no matter how many hormones they prescribe. I can replace the hormones that decline with age—that's the easy part. But there's one hormone I can't control. The good news: *you* can.

By understanding how you can control this hormone, you'll learn when you can eat all the calories you want and not get fat, and when you really need to watch the calories. You'll never have to be hungry and your fat loss will be effortless. You will be healthier, have more energy, and live longer. The second part of your life can be more vibrant and fulfilling than the first.

Let me show you how.

Jeffrey S Dunham

Jeffrey S. Dunham, M.D., Ph.D., M.P.H.
Medical Director, BioFit Medical Group

Part One

UNDERSTANDING
THE LOW-GLYCAL DIET

CHAPTER 1

WHY WE GET FAT—
IT'S NOT WHAT YOU'VE BEEN TOLD

Mauritania is one of the poorest nations on earth. Situated at the western edge of the Sahara Desert, approximately three-quarters of the land is desert or semi-desert, and most of the population farms or raises livestock for a living. It periodically suffers from severe, extended droughts and has one of the lowest GDP rates in Africa. There are no fast-food restaurants in the country, not even in the capital, Nouakchott. No Dunkin' Donuts, Big Macs or Big Gulps. There are no processed foods loaded with high-fructose corn syrup, no Cheetos or Cheez-Its. Yet Mauritania has an obesity problem. About one-fifth of the women in this impoverished country are obese and at least one-half are overweight.

Why should any of this matter to you? It matters because in Mauritania women manage to get fat without the usual suspects. Most "experts" will claim that the current obesity epidemic is a result of the overabundance and availability of calorie-dense, nutrient-poor processed foods combined with sedentary lifestyles, which is typical of most modern societies. But is that really the reason? Could the situation in Mauritania offer important insights into the real causes of obesity? How is it possible for Mauritanian women to gain all that weight in a poverty-stricken environment?

The answer is in part cultural, but ultimately stems from what these women eat. In Mauritania, fat is beautiful. Poems and love songs dating back to the 11th century glorify the obese woman, immobilized by fat, and completely dependent upon a man to hoist her up onto a camel. Obesity is a sign of wealth; thin is a sign of poverty. A young girl must be obese to be attractive to men and acceptable for marriage. So, mothers take their daughters, some as young as eight years old, to fat camps and force-feed them until they're obese. If a girl refuses to eat, the older women squeeze her feet with pincers, pinch her inner thighs or bend her fingers backwards. If a girl vomits, the women will force her to eat her own vomit.

This technique or "gavage," derived from the French term for force-feeding geese whose livers will be made into a pâté called foie gras, has been honed over a thousand years to get young girls as fat as possible, as quickly as possible. It's *The Biggest Loser* in reverse. And remember, these are young girls, not post-menopausal women. They have high levels of growth hormone, the body's most important fat-burning hormone. It's hard to get a young girl fat, but in Mauritania it's an art. So how, in this impoverished place, do they do it?

Well, let's take a look at their diet.

Breakfast consists of bread crumbs and olive oil, accompanied by high-fat camel milk. Lunch is pounded millet mixed with butter, and more milk. A young girl may eat two or three lunches a day. All told, she may drink up to 20 liters of high-fat camel milk and eat two kilograms of ground millet mixed with two cups of butter, every day. In other words, her meals are half fat, half carbohydrate, with a sprinkling of protein from the milk. This, it turns out, is the perfect recipe for a poor man's weight-gain program. What is it about this diet that is making these women obese? Is it simply the amount of food eaten, or is there something about the combination of fat and carbohydrate in the meals that is particularly fattening? In terms of the macronutrient composition of each meal (fat, protein and carbohydrate), as we'll learn later, most Americans are eating exactly the same thing, and they don't even know it. Could it be that this combination—half fat, half carbohydrate—is the cause of *our* current obesity epidemic?

If you're reading this book, you've probably tried other diets and failed. Maybe you've failed because the diet just didn't work for you, despite following it to a "t." Maybe it had too many rules, making it difficult to follow. Or maybe you had some success initially, but were unable to maintain it because the diet was too restrictive, excluding many of the foods you enjoy, making it impossible to follow for life.

With so many diets out there, how do you decide on the best one? That was the goal of a recent study published in *The Journal of the American Medical Association* on September 3, 2014. Researchers from McMaster University and the Hospital for Sick Children Research in Toronto examined data from 48 randomized clinical trials of diets including Atkins, South Beach, Zone, Biggest Loser, Jenny Craig, Nutrisystem and Weight Watchers. After some complicated statistical analysis, the researchers concluded: *any diet will work if you just stick with it.* I had to laugh when I read it. Is that the best medical science can offer to help curb the obesity epidemic? Is that what I'm supposed to tell my patients when they ask me the best way to lose weight: Just pick a diet and stick with it? Thanks for the non-answer. It reminded me of the time I asked a friend of mine who had made a fortune buying and selling real estate how he did it. His answer: "It's easy; first you have to get a job that pays really, really well."

What, then, makes a diet work? In order for a diet to work it must:

1. Be scientifically sound and make physiological sense, which means if you do follow it, you will lose weight.

2. Be easy to follow.

3. Be one you are able to maintain for life.

Let's take a look at some of the most popular diets and see if they meet the criteria to be successful.

THE LOW-FAT, CALORIE-RESTRICTED DIET

Calorie-restricted diets are usually also low fat, since there are twice as many calories in a gram of fat than a gram of protein or carbohydrate. They typically revolve around counting calories. You track the calories you eat; you track the calories you burn. The difference determines the number of pounds lost or gained, based on 3,500 calories equaling one pound of fat. Proponents of calorie-restricted diets tell you that if you can create a calorie deficit of just 100 calories a day (36,500 calories a year), you'll lose approximately 10 pounds of fat in one year. That's the generally accepted strategy for weight loss.

And it's total nonsense.

First of all, it's true that if you have a calorie deficit you'll lose weight, but it's not going to be all fat. Some of it is going to be muscle. And since there are only about 600 calories per pound of muscle tissue (70 percent of muscle is water), if your weight loss came only from muscle, you'd lose about 60 pounds of muscle in that same year—obviously not a good thing. So, what determines whether the weight loss is fat or muscle when you restrict calories? What happens during extreme calorie restriction—starvation—holds important answers.

G.F. Cahill Jr. and his colleagues at Harvard Medical School worked out the details of starvation's effects about 45 years ago. They found that when they starve normal males (all had volunteered for the study), a particular sequence of events ensues. First, the body devours the sugar stores (glycogen) in the liver and muscles for energy. Since each gram of stored glycogen carries about four grams of water with it, most of the initial weight loss is water. About two days into the fast, the subcutaneous and abdominal fat start to burn. This happens just as the glycogen stores are running out. Now, theoretically, for a normal 150-pound male, there's enough energy stored in fat to last for three months. But, before the end of the third day, the body starts breaking down muscle!

Why is muscle cannibalized so soon if there's so much fat around? The answer lies in the fact that the brain uses mainly sugar (glucose) for fuel. Under resting conditions, this can be about 20 percent or more of the total energy supply. If the blood glucose level drops too low, severe neurological disturbances take place. The liver can't make the needed glucose by breaking down fat (triglycerides), but it can from protein. So, the body attacks the muscle to save the brain. This is why calorie-restricted diets result in muscle loss as well as fat loss.

But, you *will* lose weight on a calorie-restricted diet. So the first criterion listed above is satisfied.

Are calorie-restricted diets easy to follow?

Let's take a look at the American Heart Association Diet. This diet has been around since the 1970s, and is the diet that most physicians advise their patients to follow. This diet recommends that you, "Start by knowing how many calories you should be eating and drinking to maintain your weight," and, "Don't eat more calories than you know you can burn up every day." And if you do, "Increase the amount and intensity of your physical activity to match the number of calories you take in."

Sound easy enough? Well, it sounds like a lot of weighing and calculating is involved. First you need to know how many calories you burn in the resting state, that is, your basal metabolic rate. There's a formula for it based on age, sex, height and weight, so you'll need a calculator. Then you'll need to estimate how many calories you burn in excess of your basal metabolic rate, which depends on your activity level. Are you sedentary, lightly active, moderately active, very active or extremely active? Once you get all these numbers down you need to start weighing out your food to calculate how many calories you're taking in.

I think you get the idea: It's impossible to follow.

Weight Watchers®, another calorie-restricted diet, makes it easier to follow by assigning points to foods based on nutritional content, and requires you to stick to your daily "Points Plus target," a number based on your sex, weight, height and age. It allows you to eat any food, so in this respect it's a more realistic diet. You're still able to indulge yourself with your favorite foods, as long as you don't exceed your allotted daily points. But that's the sticking point: Portions are small so you'll never really be satisfied. You're encouraged to fill up with fruits and vegetables, but how realistic is that? Support is available in the form of optional weekly meetings. And that's a good thing. You'll need all the support you can get because you'll always be tired and hungry.

And that's the Achilles heel of calorie-restricted diets: They increase hunger, so they're difficult to maintain long-term. The secretion of leptin, the hormone that tells your brain to stop eating, plummets as soon as you start restricting your calories, so you're hungry from the start. And if you're continually taking in fewer calories than you're burning, you'll *always* be tired and hungry. If you can tolerate this, you'll lose some weight initially. But your body will try to adjust to the calorie restriction by burning fewer calories. You'll secrete less thyroid hormone, the hormone that determines how many calories your cells burn. In other words, you'll become relatively hypothyroid and your metabolism will slow down. But if you want to continue to lose weight, you'll have to take in even fewer calories since your body is burning fewer calories. You'll continue this downward spiral until you just can't take it anymore and go back to eating the way you did before. And because your thyroid hormone levels have dropped and you're burning fewer calories per day than you were before the calorie restriction, you'll gain back all the weight you lost and then some.

When that happens, you'll feel like a failure. You'll feel that you have some defect in your character that makes you unable to control your eating. You'll feel terrible about yourself and search for help. You'll start going to meetings again. Maybe you'll lose the weight again, but you'll never be able to keep it off. Like a roller coaster, your weight will go up and down, over and over, year after year. Each time your weight comes back you'll think it's your fault and make up some excuse, but you've been set up for failure from the get-go.

Kirstie Alley, spokesperson for Jenny Craig, another low-fat, low-calorie diet, lost 75 pounds from 2004 to 2007, only to gain all of it back. According to Fox Business, weight-loss companies pay their celebrity spokespersons an average of $33,000 per pound of weight loss. If that can't keep you cutting calories, nothing will.

So how do calorie-restricted diets score on the criteria I outlined above? They *do* work to lose weight, but it's not all fat; you'll lose muscle too. Some of these diets are easier to follow than others; but they're all impossible to maintain for life. Strike three.

Yet most people still resort to calorie-restriction when they want to lose weight. They think that when they eat more calories than they burn, they'll store those excess calories passively as fat and, conversely, if they eat fewer calories than they burn, they'll lose that fat. But nothing happens passively in the body. Hormones drive fat storage, just like most physiological processes in the body. *And insulin is the main driver of fat storage.* You can't store fat without it.

When a child develops type-1 diabetes, for example, he stops secreting insulin and starts losing weight. His concerned parents may try feeding him more calories. But the child will continue to lose weight until a doctor makes the diagnosis of type-1 diabetes and prescribes the necessary insulin injections. Only then will the child start to gain back the weight he's lost. Insulin is necessary to get sugar (glucose) into the cells of the body. Without it, you lose weight and eventually die. But if you have too much insulin, it drives those excess calories into fat, making you fat *and* increasing your risk of type-2 diabetes, heart disease, cancer and dementia.

Insulin also drives sugar into muscle and liver cells, but both tissues have a limit as to how much sugar they can store as glycogen (the storage form of glucose). Once the maximum amount of sugar is stored as glycogen, insulin will drive the excess sugar into fat. Fat, unlike muscle or liver, can store unlimited amounts of sugar as fat. The fat cells get bigger and bigger as they store fat, and, as a result, you get fatter and fatter.

And what causes you to secrete insulin? Your pancreas secretes insulin in response to a rise in blood sugar. The faster the blood sugar rises, the more insulin it releases into the blood. And what causes your blood sugar to rise? Only carbohydrates raise blood sugar. Eating protein or fat by itself won't budge it, unless you eat huge amounts of protein at once. In that case, the excess protein converts to sugar in your liver and, indirectly, raises your blood sugar level. This is why carbohydrates are necessary to store fat.

THE LOW-CARBOHYDRATE DIET

Now that you know that carbohydrates are necessary to store fat, you can understand the underlying principles of low-carbohydrate diets. The Atkins Diet is the most well-known and studied low-carbohydrate diet. While Dr. Atkins recognized insulin as "the fat-producing hormone," he didn't make the distinction between "good" carbs and "bad" carbs. Patients could eat all the meat, chicken, seafood and eggs they wanted; as long as they avoided carbohydrate-containing foods like bread, cereal, pasta, fruits and some vegetables.

When Dr. Atkins started putting his overweight cardiac patients on this diet in the 1970s, the medical establishment viciously attacked him and labeled him a quack. They claimed that he was causing heart attacks by recommending such a high-fat diet. The consensus medical opinion at the time was that fat made you fat, and increased your risk of heart disease, even though there wasn't much evidence to support it.

But it turns out that Dr. Atkins' critics were wrong on both counts. During the past 10 years there have been a plethora of medical studies supporting the thesis that carbohydrates, not fat, make you fat. And the latest studies show no correlation between saturated fat in the diet and risk of heart disease. Unfortunately, Dr. Atkins died before his vindication.

So do low-carbohydrate diets like the Atkins Diet work? Yes, you'll lose weight if you dramatically restrict the carbohydrates in your diet. Are they easy to follow? Yes and no. Since you can eat unlimited amounts of carbohydrate-free foods like meat and cheese, and some very low-carbohydrate vegetables, no weighing is involved and it's easy to do. But eliminating all carbohydrates from your meals at home and dinners out is difficult. And it's impossible to maintain for life.

THE LOW-GLYCEMIC INDEX DIET

It turns out that you don't need to avoid all carbohydrates in your diet to keep insulin levels low; there are good carbs, bad carbs and borderline carbs. The faster the carbohydrates you consume are absorbed, the faster your blood sugar level goes up, and the more insulin you secrete. And since it's insulin that causes you to store fat, you can minimize fat storage by simply avoiding foods that spike your blood sugar.

An example of a good carbohydrate is a fresh apple; a bad carbohydrate is a slice of white bread. They both have carbohydrates. The apple has fructose (a form of sugar); white bread has starch, which converts quickly to glucose after it is absorbed. But there's not a lot of digestion required when you eat a piece of white bread. You almost begin digesting it when you put it in your mouth. The apple, by contrast, requires a certain amount of digestion to release the sugar. You chew it up, it's ground up and liquefied in your stomach, and the sugar is absorbed slowly as it moves through your small intestine. So white bread spikes your blood sugar resulting in an insulin surge that drives a significant portion of the calories in the bread into fat cells. The apple causes the blood sugar to rise more slowly, resulting in less insulin and less fat storage.

The measure of how fast 50 grams of available carbohydrate (total carbohydrates minus fiber) in a food raises your blood sugar is the glycemic index (GI) of that food. It is an experimentally determined number, calculated by measuring the blood sugar rise in volunteers after they consume 50 grams of available carbohydrate in a particular carbohydrate-containing food. The GI of a food ranges from 0 to 100, where 100 is pure glucose. The GI of white bread is 70; a fresh apple is 38. Dr. David Jenkins developed the concept of glycemic index in the early 1980s, during his research to find the best foods for diabetics. This was well after Dr. Atkins published his book, *Dr. Atkins Diet Revolution,* in 1972.

It turns out that the form of the food, how fast it's absorbed and its carbohydrate content are all critical when it comes to fat storage. You can have two foods that have the same number of calories and the same number of carbohydrates, but one will be more fattening if it's absorbed faster. Have you ever heard the expression, *"Eat the fruit; don't drink the juice?"* When you eat a fresh apple, the sugar is absorbed slowly, so you don't get a rapid rise in blood sugar and a big insulin surge. But when you juice the apple, you've already done the digestion in your juicer. What remains is basically sugar water, which is very quickly absorbed and spikes your blood sugar, resulting in an insulin surge.

Most foods in their natural state (fresh fruit, vegetables, legumes and nuts) have a relatively low GI. Processed carbohydrates, by contrast, tend to have a high GI. Foods you have to cook for a long time before you eat them generally will have a high GI by the time they're fully cooked. For example, if you were to eat a raw potato, it would be hard to digest, so the GI would be low. But when you cook it at 400°F (200°C) for an hour and make it all nice and fluffy, it's quickly absorbed and easily digested, so its GI goes up to 85. Similarly, you can't eat raw white rice, but when you cook it the GI is 98. If you eat pasta "al dente," it's less fattening than if it's overcooked. It's the same pasta, but the form is different (firm versus mushy).

Bottom line: *the form of the carbohydrate is the critical variable. The faster it's absorbed, the fatter you get.*

One of the most popular low-GI diets is the *South Beach Diet*, which is easier to follow than the Atkins Diet since it allows you to eat more carbohydrate-containing foods, as long as they have a low GI. But it still restricts high GI foods like pasta, bread, rice, potatoes and some fruits, so it requires considerable effort to follow indefinitely. This is the diet that I initially recommended to my patients 12 years ago when I started my anti-aging practice in Palm Springs. There is no weighing, so you can eat as much as you like of the low-GI foods like meat, cheese, vegetables and nuts. And since adding fat to carbohydrates in a meal slows the absorption of those carbohydrates, having a little fat with your carbs should, according to proponents of *The South Beach Diet*, result in less insulin and less fat storage.

Dr. Agatston, author of *The South Beach Diet*, advises "A little olive oil on your bread, or some low-fat cheese, is actually better for you than the bread alone." He also goes on to say, "Believe or not, that baked potato will be less fattening topped with a dollop of low-fat cheese or sour cream. The calorie count will be slightly higher, but the fat contained in the cheese or sour cream will slow down the digestive process, thereby lessening the amount of insulin that potato prompts your body to make."

But this aspect of the diet never made sense to me and, as I found out very quickly, didn't work for my patients. The baked potato with toppings has more calories but *is* more slowly absorbed, producing less insulin. But there are more calories (in the form of fats and sugars) in the blood for insulin to drive into fat cells. At what point do the added calories make up for the drop in insulin with respect to fat storage? Can you really eat all you want of low-GI foods and still lose fat?

I follow my patients very closely. At each visit I ask them what they've been eating, and measure their body fat percentage with the Bod-Pod®, the state-of-the-art method for analyzing body composition. It became apparent to me that my patients who ate an entire jar of cashews every afternoon because I told them that nuts have a low GI, or patients who tried to lower the GI of their potato by smothering it with butter and sour cream, weren't losing any fat.

I also found that patients who didn't eat breakfast or skipped lunched and had a big dinner, weren't losing fat even though their dinner contained mostly low-GI foods. These patients usually had very demanding jobs and worked long hours. They ate dinner late, and usually continued snacking until bedtime. The snacks were also low GI: nuts, cheese and occasional low GI fruits like berries or apples. But there was no fat loss. There was something about eating a large amount of food all at once, even if the foods were low GI, which prevented fat loss. Similarly, snacking on low-GI foods late at night and especially before bed made fat loss impossible.

I remember one patient in particular (I'll call him Rob), who wasn't losing fat even though at each visit I went through his diet to make sure he was truly eating only low-GI foods. Rob described the same diet at every visit: bacon and eggs for breakfast, an apple midmorning, a salad with chicken or fish for lunch, cashews and cheese in the afternoon, meat and vegetables for dinner, with occasional fruit for dessert. All low-GI foods, but yet there was no fat loss. I would see Rob about every six months. Finally at one visit, the Bod Pod showed he had dropped four percentage points in body fat. I asked him what changed and he told me he eliminated the cashews and cheese in the afternoon and ate more fruit like watermelon and apples. Now, watermelon has a GI of 72, and apples a GI of 38. The cashews and cheese he gave up have a GI of 22 and 0, respectively. He gave up some low-GI foods, substituted higher GI foods, and finally lost fat. Obviously the low-GI diet I had recommended was not working for him.

So how do low-GI diets fare with respect to the three principles necessary for a weight-loss diet to work? Well, they're easier to follow since there is no weighing involved and patients can eat as much as they'd like as long as the foods have a low GI. Patients also seem to be able to maintain them better than low-carbohydrate diets since they're able to eat more carbohydrate-containing food. But in my experience, they didn't work for everyone.

When I started to see more patients like Rob—diligently following a low-GI diet but not losing fat—I began to think more about the diet I was recommending. Nuts and cheese have a lot more calories than fruit, although the GI is much lower. Could that have something to do with it? How did calories enter into the picture? What's more important, calories or the GI values? Was there a diet that could take both into account? Would that diet produce better results? I wanted to know, and decided to do some research.

I found out that the GI (glycemic index) of a food is not a very useful number after all. As we learned earlier, the GI of a food is the measure of how fast 50 grams of available carbohydrate in a food raises your blood sugar. But this number can be deceptive. To give you an example: the GI of watermelon and white rice are both high, so, you might think it's best to avoid both of these foods. But in order to get 50 grams of *available* carbohydrate in rice you'd need to eat just a half a cup. For watermelon, since most of the weight is water, you would need to eat about two pounds to get 50 grams of *available* carbohydrate. So you're really not comparing equal serving sizes of the two foods when using the glycemic *index.*

When you adjust for serving size you get the *glycemic load,* which is a more accurate way to predict whether a food or combination of foods in a meal will cause fat storage and weight gain. To calculate the glycemic load (GL) of a food, you take into account *how much* of it you eat in a serving. The GL of a food measures how fast a normal-sized serving of that food raises blood sugar. When you look at the GL of *one* serving of watermelon, it's actually quite low, while the GL of *one* serving of white rice is still high. Thinking in terms of GL, one serving of watermelon does not spike your blood sugar and cause an insulin surge, while one cup of white rice does. This means watermelon *is* acceptable—not what you would think if you were deciding what to eat strictly on the basis of the GI.

This can be a confusing point but it's important: there is a distinction between glycemic index and glycemic load and understanding that difference is the key to losing fat effortlessly, without avoiding some high-GI foods like cantaloupe, grapes and watermelon. The total glycemic load of your meal measures how fast that particular meal will raise your blood sugar. This in turn determines how much insulin you secrete, and, consequently, how much fat you'll store from that meal. But don't worry if this is sounding complicated—at the end of the day, you'll just need to follow the simple color-coded recipes in Part Two of this book.

It's instructive to take a look at the glycemic load of different categories of food. When comparing foods with respect to glycemic load, however, we must use the same amount of food, so all of the following GL values are for 100-gram servings.

If we look at the category of "Meat, Chicken, Seafood and Eggs," we see that these foods have no carbohydrates. If they have no carbohydrates, they can't raise your blood sugar, so the GL must be 0.

FOOD	TYPE	GL (100 g)	NET CARBS (100 G)
Bacon	fried	0	0
Beef	burger, grilled	0	0
Chicken	breast, meat and skin	0	0
Eggs	scrambled	0	0
Tuna	canned, in oil	0	0

You could eat as much of these foods as you like and, if that's all you ate, insulin levels would drop and you'd lose weight, just like children when they develop type-1 diabetes.

A serving of most cheeses will have a GL of 0 as well because, when you make cheese, the bacteria ferment the milk sugar (lactose) out of the final product. What remains is solely protein and fat. So, if there are no carbohydrates, the GL again must be 0. You could eat as much meat and cheese as you like and you'd lose fat. That's basically the Atkins Diet!

FOOD	TYPE	GL (100 g)	NET CARBS (100 G)
Cheese	cheddar	0	0
Cheese	Colby Jack	0	0
Cheese	cottage, regular	0	0
Cheese	mozzarella	0	0
Cheese	Swiss	0	0

Carbohydrate-containing foods in their natural state, like fresh fruits, vegetables and nuts, have a low GL. A fresh apple has a GL of 4, while a handful of blueberries has a GL of 5. A slice of fresh pineapple has a GL of 7. But remember, we're dealing with a single serving of pineapple. So if one slice has a GL of 7, two slices have a GL of 14, three slices 21, and so on. Even if you're eating low-GI foods like fruit, if you eat too much at once you'll still spike your blood sugar.

FOOD	TYPE	GL (100 g)	NET CARBS (100 G)
Apple	fresh	4	11
Banana	fresh, ripe	12	23
Blueberries	fresh	5	12
Pineapple	fresh	7	10
Strawberries	fresh	2	6
Watermelon	fresh	5	7

Vegetables, nuts and soy contain fewer carbohydrates than fruit, so they generally will have an even lower GL. A baked potato is the exception since it has more net carbs, and cooking it for an hour at 400°F (200°C) makes it easily absorbed and digested.

FOOD	TYPE	GL (100 g)	NET CARBS (100 G)
Asparagus	steamed	0.5	1
Avocado	raw	0.5	2
Broccoli	steamed	0.5	1
Peanuts	dry roasted	1	10
Potatoes	baked	27	32
Soy Beans	cooked	1	5
Tomatoes	raw	1	3
Walnuts	plain	1	7

The real problem, however, is the category of "Breads, Pasta, Pastries and Grains." Some of the cereals you see advertised as health foods actually have some of the highest GL values. Cheerios has a GL of 60; Rice Krispies, which almost dissolve in your mouth when you eat them, has an even higher GL of 76. These cereals have a high number of net carbs per serving, and are among some of the most fattening foods that you can eat, despite the manufacturer's health claims.

FOOD	TYPE	GL (100 g)	NET CARBS (100 G)
Bread	white	34	49
Bread	whole wheat	32	42
Breakfast Cereals	Cheerios	60	81
Breakfast Cereals	Rice Krispies	76	93
Pasta	fettuccine	19	47
Rice	white	30	31

REMEMBER THIS: whole grains are good for you if you eat the whole grain, like whole-grain steel-cut oats or flax seeds, which have a very low GL. Although these foods contain carbohydrates, they're hard to digest and are absorbed slowly. Consequently, the blood sugar rise is gradual and the insulin surge minimal, resulting in less fat storage. When you pulverize the grain to make flour, however, you increase the surface area and change the rate of absorption from slow to fast. So, anything made with flour—like bread, baguettes, bagels and pasta—will have a high GL. And grains that you have to cook for a long time to eat, like rice, will usually have a high GL by the time they're ready to eat. It's the processing of food that's made it fattening. I tell my patients if they see foods advertised as "made from whole grains," they should avoid them, since it means they're highly processed. I also tell them to avoid low-fat or fat-free foods, since food manufacturers have taken the fat out of foods and replaced it with sugar to make them more palatable. This advice generally goes against everything they've been told.

But glycemic load is only part of the story. *Calories count too.* How calories interact with glycemic load is the other part of the equation. The next chapter will introduce the "glycal," which depends upon both glycemic load *and* calories, and is a *much* more accurate measure of how fattening a meal will be. By the time you finish reading the first two chapters of this book, I promise you, you'll understand the concept. You'll "get it" and be able to jump into the 3-step action plan laid out in Part Two of this book.

Let's go!

CHAPTER 2

HOW TO LOSE WEIGHT WITHOUT BEING HUNGRY—

INTRODUCING THE GLYCAL

UNDERSTANDING HOW WE GET FAT
AND THE ROLE OF HORMONES

During my summers in Boston, where I spent most of my twenties, I often drove out to Cape Cod. The long, sandy beaches, miles of dunes and fresh sea air were exactly the tonic I needed to recharge from the stresses of medical school. But escaping the city for a weekend on the Cape was never that easy for me; the trip was long, traffic was usually horrendous and the route required navigating through three rotaries on the way to my destination. Being from Chicago—where the city is a grid of blocks with stop signs and stop lights—I had never encountered a traffic rotary, and found using them a bit nerve-wracking. In Chicago, I could travel from one end of the city to the other by driving in a straight line.

When I first started driving in Boston, I was constantly getting lost because it was impossible to go any distance without hitting a rotary, which to me seemed like a manic free-for-all. Three or sometimes four roads would converge at the edge of the circle; the cars would enter and drive around it counterclockwise with the goal of exiting the circle at another point, accessing another road. But figuring out which road to take to get out of the circle was tricky. Cars would dart from the inner lane of the rotary to make their exit, cutting off other cars. Horns blared and tires screeched—a total mess.

On one of my trips to the Cape, I discovered a great little seafood restaurant, Sandy's, located off the rotary near the base of the Bourne Bridge. I particularly remember the clam chowder: fresh clams, seawater from inside the clams, cream and butter. I almost always tried to make a stop at Sandy's but only managed to find it about half the time. Frequently, I'd exit off the rotary on the wrong road and end up going miles in the wrong direction before I realized it. It was frustrating. I never really got the hang of that rotary.

Why am I telling you a story about rotaries? Because how you use the calories you eat is similar to a car traveling down a road and through a rotary. Think of the calories in a meal as passengers in cars (food) traveling down a thoroughfare (your esophagus), approaching a rotary (your stomach) with three roads radiating out from it. Inside the rotary is a traffic cop using signals (your hormones) to direct the cars toward one of the three roads. When thyroid hormone levels are high, the cop directs the cars down one road where they crash and burst into flames, burning the calories and releasing the energy needed for the body to meet its basal metabolic requirements. When testosterone and growth hormone levels are high, the cop guides the cars down another road leading towards a construction zone where the calories provide the fuel for the growth of muscle and lean body mass. But when insulin levels are high, the cop orders the cars to drive directly down a road leading into a large parking lot (fat cells) where the calories sit and wait until needed by the body.

The cars come in three models: fat, protein and carbohydrate. Each time you eat during the day, the cars carrying the calories create a kind of rush hour where the roads fill up. At this time the traffic cop has to be extra vigilant in directing the traffic. If some of the cars are carbohydrates that spike your blood sugar and raise your insulin level, the cop begins diverting cars and the calories they contain into the parking lot (fat cells) until traffic starts to move again. At night, when you stop eating and the incoming traffic slows to a trickle, the cars in the parking lot are finally able to exit and travel down the roads leading to energy (to keeping your body running through the night), and lean body mass (where the calories provide the fuel to build muscle or repair damage to your vital organs). Translation: we store fat during the day when we're eating and generating insulin, and we burn fat at night while we sleep and insulin levels drop.

The sex hormones (testosterone and estrogen) determine where the cars park in the lot (fat stores). In men, testosterone directs the cars to the belly (visceral fat). In women, estrogen directs the cars towards the breasts, buttocks and upper thighs. After menopause, when estrogen levels drop, the cars start to migrate to the belly, just like in men.

The strength of the signals (hormones) the cop uses depends upon your age, gender, weight, body composition and the type of food you eat. Now, there's not much you can do to change your age and gender, characteristics that determine the levels of thyroid hormone, growth hormone, testosterone and estrogen. The strength of these signals will determine the number of cars traveling down the roads leading to energy and lean body mass. Since the levels of these hormones decline with age, the traffic on the roads leading towards energy and lean body mass slowly diminishes as we get older, so we have less energy and we lose muscle. In my anti-aging practice, I replace these hormones to more youthful levels, so more calories start to flow back down these roads and my patients regain their energy, stamina and muscle.

The easy part is controlling levels of thyroid hormone, growth hormone, testosterone and estrogen; I can just prescribe the correct amounts and make adjustments by measuring blood levels and seeing how my patients respond. The hard part is controlling insulin levels, which will change in response to the *type and amount* of food eaten. If you're eating a lot of processed carbohydrates that spike your blood sugar, insulin levels will rise, and the parking lot will start filling up. But the parking lot will never fill up completely; it will just get bigger and bigger to accommodate all the cars, just like the fat cells in your body.

Now that you understand how the calories you eat are ending up in that parking lot (fat cells), you can understand how to close the entrance gate to stop the flow of calories entering, and open the exit gate to let the calories flow out. High insulin levels open the entrance gate and close the exit gate, keeping the cars flowing into the parking lot and trapping them there; low insulin levels close the entrance gate and open the exit gate, stopping the flow of cars into the parking lot and allowing the ones that are there to exit. Avoiding high-GL (glycemic load) foods that spike your blood sugar will keep insulin levels down, so the entrance gate will close and exit gate will open. When cars approach the entrance gate and can't get through, they'll double-back and head down the roads leading toward energy and lean body mass. And because the exit gate has opened, the cars (carrying calories) will start leaving the parking lot and head in the same direction. In other words, you'll lose fat, gain muscle *and* have more energy to boot!

If you're eating a lot of calories at once, you'd better make sure the gate to the parking lot is closed. If it isn't, you'll get a flood of cars pouring in and your fat stores will fill up. In other words, you can eat as much as you want at a meal and, as long as the total GL is 0, insulin levels will remain low, meaning the entrance gate to the parking lot will stay closed and you won't store any calories as fat. And if you can't store those calories as fat, you'll have to use those calories for energy or lean body mass. Since foods containing only protein and fat, like meat, fish, eggs and cheese, have a GL of 0, you can eat all you want of these foods at a meal without worrying about storing fat. But once you start adding carbs to that meal, the total GL will rise and the entrance gate to the parking lot will begin to open, allowing more and more calories in to "park" and be stored as fat, and the exit gate will start to close, trapping them there.

ENTER THE "GLYCAL"

We can see how the number of calories that end up in fat depends not only upon how that meal affects your insulin level, which determines how much the entrance gate to the parking lot (fat cells) is open, but also upon how many "cars" are traveling through the rotary after a meal. We know that the amount of insulin secreted depends upon the glycemic load of the food you eat. But how does the number of calories come into play? You need insulin to force calories into fat cells, but you still need to have the calories there to store. For example, the glycemic load of a handful of cashews is 4; the glycemic load of a fresh apple is also 4. Does that mean that they're equally fattening? One serving of cashews has about 600 calories; one fresh apple has about 50. Common sense tells you that a handful of cashews must be more fattening than an apple. And they are. There's more to fat storage than just glycemic load.

So, how exactly does that work? Why are cashews more fattening than an apple? If the glycemic load of each food is the same, the blood sugar rise is essentially the same, which means the amount of insulin secreted must also be the same. *The difference is that with a handful of cashews, there are 550 more calories in the blood* (mostly in the form of fats) *for insulin to drive into fat cells.* Insulin not only drives sugar into fat cells; it also drives fat into fat cells. Going back to our rotary analogy, the entrance gate to the parking lot (fat cells) is open about the same amount. But there's a lot more traffic going through the rotary when you're eating a handful of cashews than when you're eating an apple, so more cars (and calories) end up in the parking lot.

During the last 12 years of treating overweight patients, I've developed the concept of the *"glycal,"* which I've defined as a calorie stored as fat after a meal. This, ultimately, is what's really important if you want to lose fat, not just weight. We store fat during the day when we're eating and generating insulin, and burn fat at night when we stop eating and insulin levels drop. If you want to lose fat, you need to store as few glycals as possible during the day, so you burn more glycals at night and lose net fat.

The number of glycals in a meal depends upon both the amount of insulin generated by that meal and the total number of calories in it. And since the glycemic load of the meal is really just a measure of the amount of insulin generated after that meal, the number of glycals depends upon the total glycemic load of the meal *and* the total calories in that meal. The formula to calculate glycals takes into account that when the glycemic load of the meal is 0, there is no insulin spike to sweep those calories into fat cells, so the total number of glycals in that meal is 0. As the glycemic load of the meal increases, the number of glycals increases, but never exceeds the total number of calories in the meal.

You can think of the total glycemic load of a meal as approximately the percent of the calories in that meal that will be stored as fat. So, if the total glycemic load of a meal is 0, like a meal of just protein and fat, 0 percent of the calories in that meal will be stored as fat; and the total number of glycals will be 0. This means you could eat as much protein and fat as you wanted in a meal, and as long as the meal consisted of *only* protein and fat (no carbs), you wouldn't store any of those calories as fat. The actual formula for calculating glycals also takes into account how adding fat or protein to a meal can slow the absorption of the carbs in that meal and lower the total glycemic load, so it's a little more complicated than a straight percentage. But don't worry about it, the companion app, explained in Chapter 8, does all the calculations for you.

In our example of a handful of cashews and a fresh apple, both have a glycemic load of 4, which means about 4 percent of the calories will be stored as fat. But a handful of cashews has 600 calories, while an apple has only 50. In the case of the cashews, 4 percent of 600 calories, or 24 calories, will be stored as fat; in the case of the apple, 4 percent of 50 calories, or only 2 calories, will be stored as fat. This is why a handful of cashews is more fattening than a fresh apple, even though both have a glycemic load of 4.

CALORIES COUNT WHEN YOU'RE EATING CARBS!

The Low-Glycal Diet allows you to eat as many calories as you want at a meal, as long as the meal contains no carbs. If a meal has no carbs, the total GL must be 0 and, consequently, the number of calories stored as fat (glycals) must also be 0. But how many calories can you eat if your meal has carbs and the GL is not 0? In this case, *portion size is crucial*. You'd probably think that eating two handfuls of cashews would be twice as fattening as eating one handful of cashews. Wrong. Why? Because if you double the amount of cashews you eat, you double the calories *and* you double the glycemic load. Now two handfuls of cashews have 1,200 calories and a glycemic load of 8. If the glycemic load of the meal is approximately the percent of the calories in that meal that will be stored as fat, eating two handfuls of cashews will store 8 percent of 1,200 calories, or 96 calories as fat. Remember, one handful of cashews stores 24 calories as fat, so two handfuls stores *four times as much*! So when you splurge at night and get into that bag of potato chips, and think since you've already ruined your diet, you might as well eat the whole bag, think again...

The number of glycals in a meal goes up *exponentially* with the size of the meal. That's why some people have success with portion control. You know, the ones who say they never eat a whole meal, but just graze all day. Many of these people can stay thin eating this way, even if they eat bad food at times, because eating smaller meals more frequently stores a smaller percentage of the total calories per day than eating all the calories at once.

In my practice, the patients that have the most difficult time losing fat are the ones who skip breakfast, maybe grab a protein bar or other snack for lunch, and then have a large dinner when they get home. Since the number of calories stored as fat increases exponentially with the size of the meal, eating all your calories at once will store a lot more calories as fat than if the same amount of calories were broken up into five or six smaller meals spaced throughout the day.

THE TWO-HOUR RULE

But that brings up the question: how much time must there be between meals so that this strategy works? Well, about the same amount of time that insulin sticks around after a meal, or about two hours. When you eat a meal containing carbohydrates, your insulin level initially rises from its baseline level. After the insulin allows the sugar in the blood to enter cells to meet their energy requirements, and the excess sugar to enter fat cells to be stored as fat, blood sugar levels go back to baseline. This decreases insulin secretion and insulin levels return to baseline shortly thereafter. In most people, this process takes about two hours. And since it's insulin that causes you to store fat, this means that you're starting over again with respect to fat storage every two hours.

For example, if you ate six bananas at once, you'd store about 400 calories as fat. But if you were to eat six bananas throughout the day, eating one banana every two hours, you'd store about 90 calories as fat. So you can see that if you're just counting calories, you could get into trouble. That's why Step 1 (jumpstart) of the Low-Glycal Diet allows you eat to eat as many "green" (low glycal) meals as you want each day, as long as you separate the meals by two hours.

A meal can have a very large number of calories (like bacon and eggs) and still be green if the glycemic load is low. Conversely, a green meal can have a high glycemic load, as long as the number of calories is low. *This means that if you eat high-calorie foods containing a lot of fat, you can't eat them with any carbohydrates. If you eat carbohydrates, you need to avoid eating them with fat, so the total number of calories in the meal is low.*

EATING PROTEIN AND FAT SUPPRESSES YOUR APPETITE

In the Low-Glycal Diet, there's no limit to the number of calories you can eat in a day if the glycemic load of each meal is 0. This means that you can eat all the protein and fat that you want and, as long as you don't eat any carbohydrates with it, you won't store any fat. Does this mean that you can eat 10,000 calories a day of just protein and fat and not get fat? Well, it turns out that you won't want to eat that much. If you're only eating protein and fat, the free fatty acids (the breakdown product of fats) and amino acids (the breakdown products of protein) in your blood will suppress your appetite so you won't want to eat a lot of calories.

Going back to our rotary analogy, if you're eating only protein and fat, insulin levels will remain very low and the entrance gate to the parking lot (fat cells) will stay closed, forcing the protein and fat calories to travel down the roads leading to energy and muscle. But if you're taking in calories faster than you can burn them for energy or use them to build muscle, they have nowhere to go and the roads become jammed. At this point, no more cars (containing just protein and fat calories) can enter the thoroughfare (your esophagus) because the road and rotary are at a standstill. When this happens, your appetite plummets and, even if you force more protein and fat down your throat, you'd probably vomit it back up.

University of Vermont obesity researchers Ethan Sims and Elliot Danforth demonstrated this effect in the 1980s by conducting overfeeding studies, which varied the amounts of carbohydrate, protein and fat. According to one of their collaborators, Edward Horton, now professor of medicine at Harvard Medical School, the volunteers would sit staring at "plates of pork chops a mile high," and be unable to eat the excess number of calories that the researchers were asking of them. They just weren't hungry. Danforth remarked, "I challenge anyone to do an overfeeding study with just meat. You can't do it. I think it's a physical impossibility."

The reason they weren't hungry is that they couldn't store any of those excess calories as fat, since their meal of protein and fat generated no blood sugar spike or insulin surge. Eating all that fat and protein with no place to store the excess caused their blood levels of free fatty acids and amino acids to rise, suppressing their appetite. Interestingly, when the volunteers ate a mixed diet of carbohydrates and meat, they easily consumed the excess number of calories required, some taking in as much as 10,000 calories a day. Why the sudden change? Because the carbohydrates in their diets now provided that blood sugar spike and insulin needed to put those excess calories into fat cells. Now, the extra calories they ate would be stored in fat cells, and not accumulate in the blood and suppress their appetites. In other words, the entrance gate to the parking lot would open and the insulin surge would allow those extra calories to flow in and be stored as fat.

This is why you never have to be hungry on the Low-Glycal Diet. You can eat every two hours, as long as you eat the right foods and the right combination of foods.

EATING CARBS BOOSTS YOUR APPETITE

If you're eating high-GL foods, the entrance gate to the parking lot will open, and more calories will be driven into fat cells, leaving fewer calories to be burned for energy or used to build lean body mass. When this happens, you'll have to eat *more* calories to maintain your energy level. If you don't, you'll always be tired and hungry. This is an important point: *Eating processed and starchy carbohydrates makes you hungry, so you eat more calories than you should.*

Most people will also secrete too much insulin after they eat a large carb load. When this happens, the insulin will take too much sugar out of their blood and put it into fat, leaving them with low blood sugar two hours later and making them hungry again. Did you ever feel so bloated and tired after eating a Thanksgiving or Christmas dinner that all you could do was take a nap or plop down in front of the television and watch a football game or movie? And even though you stuffed yourself, did you ever find yourself going back for more pumpkin pie two hours later? Now a typical Thanksgiving dinner with all the trimmings (turkey, gravy, stuffing, mashed potatoes, sweet potatoes, biscuits, veggies, butter and pumpkin pie) can have close to 5,000 calories. So, why would you still be hungry two hours later after eating 5,000 calories? What's that all about?

I remember watching a documentary that dramatically illustrated this point. It featured in-depth interviews with morbidly obese people in England. We've all seen these people in reality shows, like *My 600-lb Life*, or in news programs. Some are so fat that they can't get out of bed. When they need medical attention, the caregivers call the fire department to break down the wall, since they're too fat to fit through a doorway. A crane then hoists them up through the broken wall and into the ambulance. Unfortunately, this is becoming less of a rarity.

You might be wondering, "How can people get that fat?" You'd think when they got so fat they couldn't move they'd stop eating. But they don't. Why not? That's what the interviewer asked a bed-ridden, 700-pound man featured in the documentary. As he lay in bed with only a sheet covering him and fast food wrappers littered around him, he looked up and said something like, "I don't understand what's happening to me. I can eat a dozen donuts, and then two hours later, it's like I ate nothing, and I'm starving again." And the reason he was "starving" after eating close to 3,000 calories is the same reason some people go back for seconds a few hours after a Thanksgiving dinner. The insulin he secreted after eating the donuts drove too much sugar into his fat cells, making him a little fatter, and leaving him with low blood sugar two hours later. In medical terms, this is what we refer to as "rebound hypoglycemia." Unfortunately, this man was one of the worst cases.

So, how can we prevent this from happening?

The amount of insulin a person secretes after eating a standard carbohydrate-containing meal will vary depending on that person's genetic makeup. But even if you're genetically predisposed to be a high-insulin secretor, you need an environmental stimulus to turn on the genes that result in this sequence of events. And that environmental stimulus is eating a food that spikes your blood sugar. So the solution for this man isn't to eat fewer donuts at a time; the solution is to change the type of food he eats. If he switched from donuts to cheese and nuts, for example, he'd secrete much less insulin and his blood sugar would remain more even between meals, curbing his hunger.

We've seen that insulin not only makes you fat; it makes you hungry as well—a vicious cycle that can trap many people into life-long obesity. The food companies know this—processed foods that spike your blood sugar cause you to crave more processed foods. Food companies don't make money on apples; they make it on cereals, crackers, cookies and other snack foods. That's why your supermarket is loaded with these items. Processed foods are the most profitable for the food companies, and when you eat them you crave more—optimizing corporate profits at the expense of your waistline. And when you get fat and acquire all the health problems associated with it, the drug companies make huge profits—but that's another story.

THE MORE CARBS YOU EAT, THE FEWER CALORIES YOU BURN

What makes it even worse is that when you refuse to give into to those hunger pangs in an attempt to lose fat, your body tries to compensate for the lack of calories by secreting less thyroid hormone, winding down your metabolism in the process. This makes it harder and harder to keep the fat off; and you have to eat fewer and fewer calories just to maintain the fat loss. This was the conclusion of a recent study published in the *Journal of the American Medical Association*. Researchers measured the total energy expenditure (calories burned) per day in volunteers on three different diets: a low-fat, high glycemic-load diet; a moderately low-glycemic load diet; and a very low-glycemic load diet. All three diets had the same number of calories; just the *types* of calories were different. Also, the participants in each group were similar to each other with respect to age, height, weight and ethnicity. Nevertheless, the subjects on the very low-glycemic load diet (10 percent carbs, meaning minimal insulin to drive calories into fat) burned more calories per day than those on the moderately low-glycemic load diet (40 percent carbs, meaning more insulin to drive calories into fat), who burned more calories than those on the low-fat, high glycemic-load diet (60 percent carbs, meaning the most insulin to drive calories into fat). From highest to lowest, the difference was about 300 calories per day. That's equivalent to about one hour of moderate-intensity exercise!

So apparently a calorie is not *always* a calorie. In terms of our rotary analogy, the type of car (carbohydrate, protein or fat) carrying those calories determines whether or not the traffic cop will direct those calories into fat cells *and* how many calories will be left to burn for energy. More calories driven into fat cells means fewer calories left for energy. A calorie from bread is not the same as a calorie from cheese, at least from the cop's perspective. Where the calories come from matters!

True or False? People get fat because they eat too much and exercise too little. Sounds reasonable enough, but the answer is false. Actually, it's the other way around. If you're eating a diet high in processed carbohydrates, you're taking a portion of the calories consumed at every meal and sticking them into fat cells. This leaves fewer calories to burn for energy, making you hungry and tired. If you're hungry you'll tend to eat too much; and if you're tired you probably won't be going to the gym. So in reality, you eat too much and exercise too little because the food you're eating is making you fat. In other words, it's not your fault! It's the food you're eating!

WHY YOU DON'T NEED TO EXERCISE TO LOSE FAT ON THE LOW-GLYCAL DIET

We burn fat with exercise only when insulin levels are low. The reason for this stems from how insulin affects lipoprotein lipase (LPL), an enzyme found on the surface of cells throughout the body. When you eat a meal containing carbs and fat, the carbs are absorbed and quickly converted to glucose, resulting in a blood sugar spike and an insulin surge. The fats are also absorbed into the blood and transported, mainly in the form of triglycerides, to cells throughout the body for use as fuel or for storage as fat. The triglycerides are too big to get into cells, so the LPL molecules on the surface of the cell bind the triglycerides and break them down into free fatty acids, which are then small enough to diffuse into the cell to be used for energy or reassembled into triglycerides for storage.

But insulin affects LPL in different ways, depending upon the cell type. In fat cells, insulin activates LPL, resulting in more binding to triglycerides and more fat stored. In muscle cells, insulin suppresses LPL, resulting in less binding to triglycerides, and less fat burned. When you exercise after eating a meal containing carbs and fat (for example, a donut), the insulin generated from the carbs drives the fat into your fat cells *and* prevents your muscles cells from taking up the fat to burn, so they burn sugar instead. This lowers your blood sugar level, which in turn increases your appetite. If you don't want to be hungry, you'll usually end up eating the same number of calories that you just burned off with the exercise, so it's a wash in terms of fat loss!

If you want to burn fat when you exercise, you need to do it when insulin levels are very low, and after you've burned through all the glycogen (sugar stores) in your liver and muscles. Normally this won't happen unless you're a marathon runner, or if you're following a very low-carbohydrate (Atkins-type) diet that depletes your glycogen stores, *and* you're exercising first thing in the morning before you've eaten, when insulin levels are lowest.

In 2010, researchers in Belgium demonstrated this effect in a group of young, healthy men. They started the men on a diet consisting of 30 percent more calories and 50 percent more fat than they'd been eating before, and divided them into three groups. One group remained sedentary; the second group began a strenuous, mid-morning workout routine *after* breakfast; and the third group did the same exercise routine, but *before* they ate breakfast. After six weeks, the sedentary group gained an average of six pounds; the group that exercised after breakfast gained about three pounds; and the group that exercised before breakfast gained no weight. The third group also burned more fat than the other two groups. In other words, exercise in the fasted state—when insulin levels are lowest—was more effective in burning fat than exercise after eating.

We've all seen that guy in the gym who's on the treadmill for an hour a day, every day, but never loses any fat. At World Gym Palm Springs, which is located adjacent to my medical office, even some of the aerobic instructors are overweight. You'd think that if they taught five to ten classes a week, there's no way they could be fat. Yet they are, and the problem is always the diet. In terms of fat loss, diet trumps exercise every time. So when that guy in the gym gets on the treadmill in the morning, trying to burn off the donut he ate a half-an-hour earlier, the insulin surge in his blood has already swept most of the calories in that donut into fat cells, making him burn the remaining sugar in his blood and not the fat he stored by eating the donut. And to top it off his declining blood sugar level is making him "work up an appetite," so he's likely to overeat after his workout.

The Low-Glycal Diet assumes that you're not a marathoner; you're not following an extremely low-carb diet; and that you're not exercising first thing in the morning before you've had breakfast, so exercise is not a part of the diet plan. This doesn't mean that you shouldn't exercise, since exercise has tremendous health benefits (other than fat loss). Exercise is an excellent way to lower blood sugar levels, improve heart and lung function, build muscle and improve mood.

It's not the best strategy, however, for fat loss.

Yet most doctors still recommend exercise to their patients as a way to take off the excess fat. But is it inactivity that has contributed to the current obesity epidemic? The growth in the number of health clubs in this country since 1980 has exactly paralleled the rise in the obesity rate. If lack of exercise was the problem, shouldn't more health clubs have put the brakes on it?

When researchers go into the bush to study the few remaining truly hunter-gatherer tribes left on earth, they're remarkably surprised at how fit and healthy they are. There is virtually no diabetes, heart disease or cancer among them. Gary Taubes, in his book, *Good Calories, Bad Calories*, documents how tribes diverse as the Inuit in the Artic, whose diet consists primarily of caribou, fish, seal and polar bear, to the nomadic Massai in Kenya, whose diet consists entirely of milk, blood and occasionally meat from the cattle they herd, remained vigorous, lean and disease-free until they adopted more of a Western lifestyle. But once introduced into the Western world, an extraordinary sequence of events ensued: First, they got fat; then they got diabetes, then heart disease and finally cancer. So what kept them healthy in their previous isolated environments? Since their diets were so diverse, was it the physical activity of the hunt and the nomadic life-style that kept them healthy? Or was it the *lack* of something?

A recent study of the Hazda hunter-gatherers of northern Tanzania sought to answer that question. The Hazda grow no food, raise no livestock and live without rules or calendars. They live a hunter-gatherer existence that is unchanged from 10,000 years ago. Their language is interspersed with tongue clicks and glottic pops, unlike any other language. There is a sexual division of labor: Hazda men hunt game and gather honey; Hazda women pick fruit and dig edible tubers. They will eat almost anything they can kill: birds, wildebeest and zebras; they particularly love baboon.

Using some sophisticated tools that included portable respirators and wearable GPS devices, researchers calculated the average total daily energy expenditure (TEE, which is total calories burned per day), of a Hazda hunter-gatherer and compared it to the TEE of a typical Western office worker. Although the Hazda had a higher level of physical activity than individuals from Western populations, their total energy expenditures, in contrast to what you might think, were virtually indistinguishable. Yet the Hazda had lower body fat percentages than their Western counterparts. So, how could the Westerners be fatter than the Hazda if they both burned the same number of calories per day? Well, if it's not exercise, it must be diet. Westerners eat more calories per day than their Hazda counterparts, and more calories than needed to satisfy their metabolic demands.

And why do Westerners eat more calories than they need? The answer lies in the *type* of calories they eat. The Hazda represent modern-day Paleolithic humans; the foods they eat—like meat, fruit, nuts and leafy greens—have a very low glycemic load. This means that their meals don't cause much of a blood sugar spike or insulin surge. In terms of our rotary analogy, the entrance gate to the parking lot stays shut most of the time for the Hazda. Without the excess insulin to open the gate, fewer calories enter fat cells and more calories are left to burn for energy. By contrast, the Western diet has a much higher glycemic load, which means that the entrance gate to the parking lot is wide open. This means that the typical modern office worker is putting a larger percentage of the calories from each meal into fat cells, making them unavailable to burn for energy. Consequently, modern workers have to eat more calories per day than the Hazda to meet their energy needs, and are fatter because of it.

We can see from the study of the Hazda that our current obesity epidemic is not the result of a lower physical activity level than our ancestors, but rather a diet that is higher in calories and total glycemic load. As we've seen in Chapter 1, most diets focus solely on calories or glycemic index, and fail to account for glycemic load, or how glycemic load and calories interact with respect to fat storage. The Low-Glycal Diet not only takes into account calories *and* glycemic load, but also how they work in concert to store fat.

DON'T EAT WHEN THE SUN "DON'T" SHINE...

I packed on 15 pounds during my first year after medical school. That may not sound like a lot, but up to that point my weight hadn't varied since high school. It was the year of my internal medicine internship at a busy hospital in San Francisco. I was on-call in the hospital every fourth night, which meant that I worked 36 hours straight every fourth night. I don't think I ate more calories during that year; I just ate my meals when I got a chance, at odd hours. On the days I was on-call, I sometimes found myself eating dinner at ten or eleven o'clock at night, after I had finished taking care of my own patients, and all the problems that came up with the other interns' patients. When I wasn't on-call, I often didn't get home until 8:00 p.m. or 9:00 p.m. That meant that I didn't eat dinner until 9:00 p.m. or 10:00 p.m., after which I immediately fell asleep since I had to be back at the hospital by 7:00 a.m.

I found out then, first-hand, what scientific research has since proved—*when* you eat can be as important as what you eat and how much you eat. A number of recent medical studies have verified what I long ago suspected: The later you eat, the fatter you get. In 2013, researchers studied a group of early-eaters and late-eaters on a 20-week, weight-loss treatment. One group ate most of their calories at lunch, while the other group ate most of their calories at dinner. Even though the participants ate the same number of calories and the same types of food, the early-eaters lost more weight than the late-eaters. This may be part of the reason why Europeans, on average, are leaner than Americans. The main meal in Europe is lunch; in America it's dinner.

Why does eating later result in more fat storage? It turns out that the answer, again, is hormones. There is a normal circadian rhythm in the levels of hormones associated with fat storage and fat burning. Insulin levels are typically elevated during the day when we're eating and lowest at night when we're sleeping. Cortisol, which stimulates the liver to produce glucose (and activates lipoprotein lipase on fat cells, causing them to take in more fat from the blood), reaches its highest level in the morning and its lowest level at night. Levels of melatonin, the hormone that makes us sleepy, start to rise when it gets dark, but drop off if we turn on a bright light. Growth hormone, the most important hormone for fat burning, reaches its highest level right after we fall asleep at night, but is undetectable during the day. Insulin and cortisol are associated with fat storage; melatonin and growth hormone are associated with fat burning.

Eating late at night bumps your insulin level when it normally should be low; being up all night under stressful circumstances spikes your cortisol level when it should normally be low. Working all night under artificial lighting shuts off melatonin secretion and decreases growth hormone secretion. In other words, working late and eating late increases the fat storage hormones and decreases the fat-burning hormones, so we get fat, even though we're eating the same number of calories per day.

Have you ever heard the expression, "No carbs after 6 p.m.?" Many fitness professionals and nutritionists will recommend this to their clients, but have no idea why it helps with fat loss. The reason is that eating carbs late at night results in an insulin surge that trumps the fat-burning effects of growth hormone, which peaks shortly after you fall asleep at night. Insulin and growth hormone are antagonistic: Insulin makes you store fat; growth hormone makes you burn fat. Avoiding carbs late at night ensures that insulin levels are low when growth hormone levels are high, resulting in the maximum fat-burning effect while you sleep at night.

Some of my patients tell me at their initial consultation that they like to have a bowl of cereal, or, even worse, cookies and milk before bed, since it seems to help them sleep more soundly. But eating cereal or cookies before bed is probably the worst thing you can do if you're trying to lose fat, and much worse than having them in the morning. The insulin surge before bed makes you start storing fat during sleep, when you really should be burning fat. Keeping insulin levels low at night is an important part of the Low-Glycal Diet. That's why the ranges of green, yellow and red meals in the Low-Glycal Diet become stricter after 6 p.m. One banana, for example, is a green snack before 6 p.m., but a yellow one after 6 p.m.

WHY WE GET FATTER AS WE AGE

One of the most common complaints I get from my patients at their initial consultation is that they're getting fatter despite eating the same diet and maintaining the same exercise routine. "I'm eating the same thing, working out more than ever and I'm still getting fat and flabby. I don't understand what's happening to me."

Insulin levels depend upon your diet; growth hormone levels depend upon your age. Since growth hormone levels decline with age, you can eat the same diet all your life (meaning you have the same insulin level) but still get fatter and fatter as you age, since there's less growth hormone around to oppose the effects of insulin. When you're an adolescent and have high growth hormone levels, you can eat junk food and still maintain a slim physique, but after 40 you can't get away with it anymore. You have to be better and better with your diet as you age if you want to maintain a low body-fat percentage.

In my practice, I try to optimize the levels of the fat-burning hormones in my patients by prescribing the appropriate amounts and checking blood levels periodically. What I can't control is the main fat-storing hormone, insulin. That's why I devote up to an hour in the initial consultation talking about diet. As we've seen, it's much more complicated than just counting calories. Luckily, The Low-Glycal Diet™ companion app makes it simple. The app calculates the number of glycals for any combination of more than 1,000 foods, reads the time on your smart phone or tablet and gives a green, yellow or red rating for any meal. And with that tool at your fingertips, you can stay on track whether at home or eating out. I've made it simple and easy to use, so don't be afraid of the technology. Chapter 8 takes you through it step by step, explaining it in detail with examples.

WHILE YOU WERE SLEEPING...

There is a significant amount of scientific research showing that the longer you sleep, the more fat you burn. A recent study in the *Annals of Internal Medicine* showed that sleep is one of the most powerful diet tools available. Researchers compared two groups of overweight, non-smokers on a calorie-restricted diet. Each group ate the same number of calories a day, but one group slept 5.5 hours a night, while the other group clocked in at 8.5 hours a night. After two weeks, the subjects who slept 8.5 hours a night lost more fat and burned an average of *400 more calories a day* than those who slept less. They also produced less of the appetite-stimulating hormone, ghrelin, than the group that slept less, so they were less hungry when they woke up.

That's why the Low-Glycal Diet counts hours of sleep toward fat loss, and not hours of exercise. You'll see in Chapter 8, how sleeping more at night will raise the limit of how many glycals you're allowed per day if you want to be in the fat-burning zone. As discussed earlier, the Low-Glycal Diet assumes that most people will eat the same number of calories they burn off with exercise if they don't want to be tired and hungry all day, so the number of hours of exercise per day doesn't enter into the calculation for fat loss. This is in contrast to most weight-loss diets, like Weight Watchers, which calculates a Points Plus value to a number of activities, allowing you to eat more calories if you exercise more. In reality, if you're eating when you're hungry and not eating when you're not, you'll eat the same number of calories you burn off with the exercise, so there's no sense in even bothering to do the calculation. In the Low-Glycal Diet, you never have to be hungry; you just have to eat the right foods and the right combinations of foods. If you want to lose more fat, just sleep more and stress less about making the time to go to the gym!

The Low-Glycal Diet comes with one important caveat: *Drinking alcohol can slow fat loss.* I always ask my patients about their alcohol consumption because it can trump even the best low-glycal meal plan. Alcohol doesn't cause a blood sugar rise or insulin surge; its GL is 0. So, as we've learned, drinking alcohol alone (without a sugary mixer or other carbohydrate-containing food) will not cause you to *store* fat. But don't think you can drink all the alcohol you want on the Low-Glycal Diet. If you have alcohol in your blood when you go to sleep, it will prevent you from *burning* fat. It turns out that it's much easier for your body to use alcohol as fuel to keep your body running through the night than it is for your body to start breaking down fat, so you'll need to burn through all the alcohol in your blood before you start breaking down fat. Your liver can metabolize about one ounce of liquor (one standard mixed drink or one glass of wine) every hour, so if you have a glass of wine with dinner, you'll probably have burned off the alcohol before bed. But if you drink half a bottle with dinner and have two mixed drinks after, you'll still have alcohol in your blood when you're sleeping and your fat loss will slow.

If you drink, don't have more than one standard mixed drink or one glass of wine per hour, and don't drink any alcohol for at least two hours before bed.

HOW AND WHY YOU CAN STILL EAT REALLY "BAD FOOD"

A few years back, I went to the beach in San Diego with some friends. It was a gorgeous sunny day and the water was actually warm enough to swim in, which is rare in California. The beach was hard to get to; we scaled down a 400-foot cliff and then walked a long way down the beach to get to the most beautiful part. After a day of swimming—and climbing back up to the parking lot—we had worked up quite an appetite. Someone in the group said he knew of a pizza place that had an all-you-can-eat special on Sundays, so we headed there. It was an all-you-can-eat buffet, where you helped yourself to whatever you wanted from a selection of three or four different deep-dish pizzas. I started in on the supreme pizza: sausage, pepperoni, veggies and mozzarella cheese. Unlike my friends, however, I ate only the toppings, leaving a pile of uneaten crust on my plate. This was the norm for me, but it seemed strange to everybody else. After about my fifth time going up to get more, I noticed the employees and restaurant manager glaring at me and talking in a huddle. Clearly, they weren't happy about me eating the pizza without the crust; it was as if I had broken the all-you-can-eat rules.

I'm telling you this story because even though I ate the toppings from the equivalent of one extra-large pizza, I didn't store any of those calories as fat. How is that possible? It's possible because, as we've learned, you need insulin to store fat, and a spike in your blood sugar to generate an insulin surge. Eating the toppings *only* (meat, cheese and fresh vegetables) without the crust (made from flour) didn't budge my blood sugar, so I didn't store any fat. I remember feeling full and sated without feeling bloated, and not very hungry for the rest of the day.

I often hear from my patients that their only options at lunch when they're working are fast-food restaurants, so it's impossible to eat well. My answer to them is that there are still healthy options; you just need to know how to eat. For example, you can have a low-carb burger, or even a double cheeseburger. Have the two beef patties with cheese; top it with lettuce, tomato and mayonnaise. Wrap it with iceberg lettuce instead of a bun, and you've just eaten a healthy meal. Add the bun or the fries, however, and you've changed that meal from a healthy one to one that's going to make you fat. Similarly, if your only choices are wraps or sandwiches, eat the insides and not the tortilla or bread.

By knowing how to combine foods and when to eat them, you can still eat some of your favorite carbs with minimal damage. If you don't want to give up your toast and coffee in the morning you can still have it, as long as you don't eat anything else with it and you eat it at least two hours after your last meal and two hours before your next meal. For example, two slices of rye toast and a cup of coffee have approximately 131 calories and a glycemic load of 14. Now 14 is a relatively high glycemic load, but there are only 131 calories around to be stored as fat. So, as we learned earlier, you'll store approximately 14 percent of 131 calories, or only about 17 calories as fat. **If you eat "bad" carbs, eat them alone, preferably earlier in the day, and at least two hours after the last meal and two hours before the next meal.**

By the way, you can still enjoy pizza—with its crust—on an occasional basis. As you're learning, making that choice a wise one will depend on what's on the pizza, the time of day you're eating it and what else you're eating with it.

Remember the diet of those young girls in Mauritania?

"Breakfast consists of bread crumbs and olive oil, accompanied by high-fat camel milk. Lunch is pounded millet mixed with butter, and more milk. A young girl may eat two or three lunches a day. All told, she may drink up to 20 liters of high-fat camel milk and eat two kilos of ground millet mixed with two cups of butter, every day."

In other words, at each meal her diet is half fat, half carbohydrate, with a sprinkling of protein from the milk. Why is this the perfect recipe for a poor man's weight gain program? Because the fat ensures the maximum number of calories, and the carbohydrates spike the blood sugar and cause an insulin surge, driving most of those calories into fat cells. Just like the fat man in England eating his dozen donuts.

The biochemistry of fat storage is the same whether you're in a fat farm in Mauritania or a corner office in Manhattan. But by knowing a little bit about how fat is stored, you can game the system and lose fat, without being hungry or giving up some of your favorite processed foods. Along the way, your cravings will change, too, making your transition to a more healthful way of eating even easier. Added bonus: you'll be slowing the aging process.

Following the Low-Glycal Diet keeps your blood sugar level low and slows the aging process. Glucose (sugar) is like gasoline. Just as your car needs gasoline to run, your body needs glucose to fuel its energy needs. But you wouldn't keep pumping gasoline into your car once the tank is full. If you did, the spilled gasoline could blow up the entire gas station if ignited by a spark or a lit cigarette. Yet many people keep consuming glucose—in the form of processed carbohydrates—in excess of their energy needs. This excess glucose in the blood not only makes cancer cells grow faster, it also binds to proteins throughout the body, essentially "curing" the body tissues in excess sugar. These "glycated" proteins can then crosslink and trigger inflammation, adding even more fuel to the fire. When this happens in blood vessels, it increases the risk of heart attack and stroke. When it occurs in the kidney, it results in chronic kidney failure. In the eye it causes cataracts and blindness; in the brain it causes dementia. These are all well-known consequences of uncontrolled diabetes. These are also features associated with aging. On a continuum, the higher the blood sugar levels are over time, the faster "aging" occurs.

Part Two

USING THE
LOW-GLYCAL DIET

THE 3-STEP PLAN, MENUS, RECIPES,
THE COMPANION APP, YOUR TEMPLATE

CHAPTER 3

READY, SET, GO!
HOW EFFORTLESS
WEIGHT LOSS CAN
BE YOURS

Congratulations! You've made it to the action part of the book and are about to change your life in wonderful ways. The results will amaze you. And, as you learned in Chapter 2, this diet is more than an excellent way to lose weight—it also has tremendous anti-aging benefits. So, let's get started!

Any lifestyle change requires a little planning, and the Low-Glycal Diet is no exception. The good news is you do not have to head out to buy expensive supplements or track down hard-to-find foods. But you will find that taking stock of what's in your cupboards, fridge and freezer—and creating smart shopping lists—will set you up for an easy transition to low-glycal eating.

HELLO, KITCHEN!

Let's start with your cupboards. All the processed or "prepared" foods should be evaluated; you may decide to get rid of some (or all) of it right away now that you understand that processed carbohydrates activate your insulin to store fat. At the very least, make note of the foods that contain high-fructose corn syrup (you'll find that information on the label). This ingredient is one to be avoided or, better yet, *eliminated* from your diet. It has zero nutritional value and is simply a cheap ingredient added to many processed foods to appeal to American's out-of-control love of sweets.

High-fructose corn syrup creates havoc with your blood sugar levels, causing insulin spikes that trigger your body to store fat *and* accelerate aging at the cellular level. Check out the labels on boxes of cereal, jars of jam, peanut butter, so-called "power bars," cookies, candy, prepared spaghetti sauce, condiments like ketchup, bottled salad dressing—virtually any prepared food on your shelf is likely to contain high-fructose corn syrup unless you have already been avoiding it when you shop. The good news is you can find brands that do *not* contain it; peanut butter that contains nothing but peanuts and salt, for example, is readily available from major food companies. The other good news: when you change your eating habits with the Low-Glycal Diet plan, you will find that your interest in sweets diminishes. Your palate and cravings will change.

You may be surprised to learn that so-called "whole grain" foods are another potential hazard. Remember this: whole grains *are* good for you IF you eat the whole grain. Flax seeds, steel cut oats, farro, wheat berries—all of these can be a tasty and healthful part of a low-glycal meal plan. Once they are processed, however—into instant cereal, crackers, bread and so on—they jump to high-glycal. That's because the milling process changes a slowly digested complex carbohydrate food into one that is much more quickly digested by your body. It takes much longer for cooked wheat berries, for example, to be digested than a piece of whole wheat bread. The longer it takes your body to digest a complex carbohydrate, the less effect that food has on your insulin levels, which in turn means less (or no) storage of calories as body fat.

That said, bread and even cookies can still be part of your diet once you've achieved your ideal weight, if you consume them following the Low-Glycal Diet plan. I find many people actually lose their desire for these items once they start eating the low-glycal way, but it's nice to know that you can indulge in treats when the desire or occasion arises without undoing all the good of the low-glycal plan.

In your fridge and freezer, in addition to watching out for high-fructose corn syrup and processed foods, look for labels that claim "low-fat" or "fat-free." These foods will *not* help you; as you have learned, it is carbohydrates, *not fat*, that cause the release of insulin and storage of calories as fat. Plus, real naturally occurring fats in foods are good for you. Also, they help you feel sated, or full, faster. When it comes to the refrigerated cases at the supermarket, you are better off to buy "whole foods," and that includes real butter (not a fat-free substitute), whole-milk yogurt (unsweetened), real cheeses and so on.

Some cheeses, such as goat's milk cheese and sheep's milk cheese, have a lower fat content naturally, so the label may shout "Low-Fat!" in bold print. These cheeses are still a good choice for you, however, because the product is a real (not reformulated) food and its low-fat profile is not due to any sort of processing. Goat- and sheep-milk cheeses are also lower-calorie than some of the cow's milk cheeses and, since calories still count in the Low-Glycal Diet, you may want to try them if you never have. Many of the recipes in this book call for them, and you'll find they make a nice addition to your meals or snacks.

CLEAN SWEEP

As you evaluate the food you have on hand, you may find yourself thinking, "Sure, that's a high-glycal item, but eventually I'll get to the point where I can eat it again, once I've achieved my weight-loss goal. So, why not keep it?" My answer: you don't need unhealthy foods around that may tempt you during Step 1 and Step 2 of the diet, so get rid of them.

It's true that the Low-Glycal Diet is designed to allow you to include "yellow" (medium-glycal) meals and even "red" (high-glycal) meals on occasion, which is why you'll stick with it. But you're about to start Step 1 now, which is all "green" (low-glycal) meals for two weeks. Give yourself the benefit of a clean start. It's worth it: During this phase you can expect to lose five to ten pounds, without experiencing hunger. Your body will thank you! And, before long, low-glycal food choices and meal preparation will be second nature.

GETTING STARTED

During Step 1, you will be eating only low-glycal meals and snacks for 14 days, which will kick-start your weight loss. The next chapter includes suggestions for what you can eat for breakfast, lunch, dinner and snacks each of those 14 days. We've put together a selection of dishes that are easy to shop for, easy to prepare and that fit the definition of "delicious!" for most people. But, if there's an item here you don't like to eat, not to worry: you'll find more than enough choices to get you through. You can also vary the day-to-day sequence of the meals to suit your schedule and tastes.

After you complete Step 1—the 14-day period of low-glycal meals and snacks that kick-starts your weight loss—you will move on to Step 2, which allows you to continue losing weight but on a plan that gives you more food choices. You'll stay on Step 2 until you reach your desired weight. Then, you graduate to Step 3, the weight maintenance plan, which has lots of flexibility and even more meal options. Each step of the diet is explained in detail in the chapters that follow.

It's easy to follow the Low-Glycal Diet way of eating. Even though the diet will likely mean changing *some* of your current eating habits—*what* you eat or *when* you eat or how *much* you eat—it won't take long for you to feel at ease with it. As a matter of fact, I think you'll find yourself wondering why everyone doesn't eat this way. You are going to feel great as you lose the excess fat and regain your energy, and you'll be enjoying wholesome meals and snacks of real foods that keep you from experiencing hunger.

The suggested meal plans and 75 recipes (including variations) in this book will help you transition to the Low-Glycal Diet way of eating. Most of the recipes create "green" (low-glycal) meals and snacks because, whether you are on Step 1, Step 2 or Step 3 of the diet, that's what most of your meals will be as you follow this plan from kick-start to maintenance. And, unless you are already using The Low-Glycal Diet companion app, we know you'll need a collection of low-glycal recipes to help you get going.

That said, you do not need to follow the meal plans "to the letter" to succeed with your weight-loss goals; you just need to keep your meals and snacks either low-, medium- or high-glycal, as the meal plans for each of the 3 steps indicate. That's it.

The menus are *suggestions* and the variety they contain is intended to show you how much flexibility the Low-Glycal Diet allows. You will determine your meals for the week to suit your tastes, budget and schedule. *Please*, do not interpret the meal plans to mean that you need to start the day with, say, a cheese omelet and bacon on Monday, oatmeal and blueberries on Tuesday, yogurt and strawberries on Wednesday—or whatever the day-to-day list suggests—for the diet to work!

BE PREPARED

You will see that each meal plan includes three meals and two snacks a day. If you have responsibilities at home and a full-time job that make you feel like you can barely get out the door on time each morning—let alone make and eat breakfast or pack a lunch—starting and following the Low-Glycal Diet will mean developing the habit of planning and preparing meals ahead. The templates in Chapter 9 will help you do that.

By keeping a smart shopping list, preparing multiple meals in advance, and keeping partially prepared recipes in your freezer, you can become a more organized, lean and youthful you.

YOUR SHOPPING CART

It's time to make a shopping list! Before you begin making a meal, or packing a week's worth of snacks for the office, you need to have all the ingredients on hand. You are getting ready to start Step 1 of the diet, so check out the meal plans that begin on page 66, and the recipes in Chapter 7 and figure out your meals for the week ahead. Once you've made your choices, make a shopping list. Now, you're ready to go. Do make sure you don't go shopping on an empty stomach. Hunger can sabotage your best intentions. This kind of weekly meal planning is important whether you are in Step 1, Step 2 or Step 3 of the diet so make it a habit now.

As you navigate the aisles of your supermarket, start with the perimeter, which is where you'll find fruits and vegetables, eggs, dairy products, meat and frozen foods. Next, find any seasoning staples you may need, such as anchovies, dried herbs, olive oil, capers and so on. Then pick up any of the non-perishable items such as steel-cut oats, walnuts, almonds and the like that are on your list. You will have in front of you a cart filled with healthful, tasty, whole foods that will make for delicious, satisfying low-glycal meals—for home or the workplace. You are ready to launch your weight loss and anti-aging plan!

STOWING THE GOODS

When you get home from grocery shopping, do you look like someone trying to set a speed-record for unloading the bags? Do you usually shove what needs to be kept cold into the fridge as fast as you can and then walk away? If so, it's time to approach this task differently. If you get in the habit of spending a *little* time preparing some of the things you've bought for the week *as you unpack them*, you'll find it easier to enjoy the Low-Glycal Diet way of eating. You'll also get the most out of your shopping dollars since items won't get "lost" in your fridge, spoiling before you notice them. Vegetables and fruits, in particular, can be cleaned and readied for a snack or to be used as an ingredient in a meal, saving you time later and ensuring that you stick to your meal plans.

FROZEN FRUITS AND VEGETABLES CAN MAKE LIFE EASY

Have bags and boxes of frozen fruits and vegetables in your freezer to help you stick with your meal plans. The nutritional value is excellent, and the convenience factor is priceless. Nowadays, the selection of frozen fruits—berries in particular—is terrific. Check the label and make sure you purchase unsweetened fruit. For vegetables, make sure they are not in a sauce; you want unadorned spinach, peas, green beans or whatever you are buying.

TAKE IT EASY!

With well-stocked cupboards and a fridge full of meats, cheeses, prepped fruits and vegetables, following the Low-Glycal Diet will be easy and delicious.

Next stop: Step 1!

CHAPTER 4

STEP 1: KICK-START THE WEIGHT LOSS—
WITH A TWO-WEEK MEAL PLAN

Welcome to Step 1 of the Low-Glycal Diet. With everything you've learned so far, you're ready to begin. During Step 1, you can expect an easy 5 to 10 pound weight loss. And you'll be losing *fat*, not muscle, without hunger. To help you get started, here is a 14-day meal plan. All the suggested meals and snacks in the plan are "green" (low-glycal), which is how you will kick-start your weight loss.

You will follow this all-low-glycal meal plan (or a modification of it based on your schedule, budget and tastes), for two weeks. During that time you will lose fat while maintaining and building lean body mass.

You should not be hungry during Step 1. By consuming three low-glycal meals a day, with low-glycal snacks in between the meals, you will be losing weight *without* hunger. This feature is an important one because hunger and the fatigue that comes with it are why so many diets don't work. During Step 1, you can eat all the meals or snacks you want as long as each meal or snack is low-glycal and is separated by two hours, *and* you do not eat after 8:00 p.m.

The Low-Glycal Diet is smart and flexible, which is why every step in the 3-step plan is do-able. Here's an example: A breakfast of an egg (prepared how you like it) with bacon or sausage is a good choice for a low-glycal meal to start your day. But, if you have a fried egg and bacon for breakfast at 7:00 a.m. and find you are hungry before a planned snack two hours later, you can adjust your meal plan to include a breakfast of two eggs with a single serving of bacon or sausage. You'll be increasing the calories a bit (by about 100) but you won't be changing the glycemic load (GL) or the glycals of your breakfast, both of which are zero in this example. In other words, you will still be eating a low-glycal breakfast and following Step 1 of the plan.

You can adjust the snacks, too, to suit your needs, as long as you keep them all low-glycal during the first two weeks on the diet. For example, if you find that a serving of dry roasted peanuts is not carrying you through between breakfast and lunch, or between lunch and dinner, you can add a serving of Cheese Sticks (check Chapter 7 for the recipe) to the serving of peanuts and still be enjoying a low-glycal snack. In this example, the GL (glycemic load) of the snack does not change (it's still 1), and the glycals only change a small amount, going from 2 glycals to 3. You can figure out the GL and glycals of any combination of foods for snacks—or any other meal—by using the free companion app, which is explained thoroughly in Chapter 8.

WHY YOU MAY BE ABLE TO HAVE EXTRA BETWEEN-MEAL SNACKS ON THE LOW-GLYCAL DIET

The meal plans in this book include suggestions for a mid-morning snack and a mid-afternoon snack every day. Keep in mind, however, that you may be able to have *two* snacks between breakfast and lunch, and/or between lunch and dinner, depending on your schedule. Here's how: If you eat breakfast at 6:30 a.m., and lunch at 12:30 p.m., you could have a snack at 8:30 in the morning (if you were hungry), and another snack at 10:30. The same holds true during the afternoon. As long as the snacks are low-glycal, and as long as you allow two hours between meals and snacks, you are still following the Low-Glycal Diet and you will be losing weight. No wonder people stick to this diet!

BREAKFAST AND SNACKS YOUR WAY

The meal plans in this chapter—and in the chapters that follow—are *suggestions.* They are intended to show you just how much variety is possible on the Low-Glycal Diet. If you are one of those people who likes to eat the same breakfast *every* day (a scrambled egg with bacon, for example), or the same mid-morning snack at the office Monday through Friday (a handful of almonds, say), that's fine! **You don't have to follow these day-by-day menus to the letter.** You simply have to ensure that during Step 1 all your meals and snacks are low-glycal and separated by two hours.

HOW TO PICTURE A SINGLE SERVING

All servings in the meal plans are "single," which are defined in the day-by-day plan or within the recipes. You will also find serving size information in the companion Low-Glycal Diet app, which you can download for free. But, you can usually picture a single serving of meat or vegetables or fruit pretty easily by thinking of it this way:

- A single serving of meat is approximately the size of a deck of playing cards
- A single serving of a vegetable is one cup, *cooked*

- A single serving of a fruit is a piece of a whole fruit (think: apple, pear, peach, banana) or a portion of it if it is large (½ a grapefruit, ¼ of a cantaloupe, a cup of grapes and so on), all of which is noted in the meal plans

The note that it's the volume of a *cooked* vegetable that is being measured for a single serving is important because most vegetables lose volume when they are cooked—some quite significantly (Swiss chard and fresh spinach are good examples).

LUNCH, YOUR WAY

The meal plans in this chapter—and in the chapters that follow—are *suggestions.* The lunch menus are intended to show you just how much variety is possible on the Low-Glycal Diet. But if you don't like to cook, or are juggling a full-time job and school and don't have time to cook, or for whatever reason find the varied menus in the meal plan overwhelming—not to worry! We know that following a diet shouldn't rule your life. You can enjoy low-glycal lunches quite simply: Keep a supply of the following go-to staples on hand and you'll be all set:

- Canned tuna (one 5-ounce [140-g] can is a single serving)

- Canned sardines (two 3.75-ounce [106-g] tins are a single serving)

- Hard-boiled eggs (1 large egg = a single serving but 2 or even 3 is still low-glycal)

- Cottage cheese (½ cup [115 g] is a single serving)

- Cheese Sticks (see page 185 for recipe)

- One serving of tuna (1 can) or sardines (2 tins) with a small green salad plus 1 serving of Cheese Sticks (or a ½ cup [115 g] of cottage cheese) is a low-glycal lunch. You can do the same with 2 hard-boiled eggs—add a small green salad lightly dressed and a serving of Cheese Sticks or a ½ cup (115 g) of cottage cheese and your low-glycal lunch awaits! (Still hungry? Have another hard-boiled egg or serving of tuna or sardines; your lunch is still low-glycal.) Enjoy (and now get back to work, or school, or those kids...)!

DINNER, YOUR WAY

The dinner menus that follow are intended to show you just how much variety is possible on the Low-Glycal Diet. But if you don't like to cook, or have very little time at the end of the day to put a meal on the table, you can get through the work week nicely enjoying satisfying low-glycal dinners quite easily: Make your go-to evening meal a single serving of meat (think: a steak, pork chop, lamb chop, cod fillet, salmon steak—you choose) plus a small green salad lightly dressed, and a serving of a steamed green vegetable like spinach or broccoli or green beans (fresh or frozen). You're done! If that isn't enough food on the plate for you, increase the serving of protein; your meal will still be low-glycal.

THE POWER OF THE PEN

Before you embark on the Low-Glycal Diet, starting with 14 days of all low-glycal meals and snacks in Step 1, take a look at the meal plan for ideas and then, using the template in Chapter 9, write down what you'll be eating. Having it in writing keeps you accountable. I suggest that you also make a photocopy of your personal meal plan and keep it where you can easily reference it during the day. Make notes on it as the days go by so that you can see what's working or where you need to make adjustments. This diet is yours; so own it!

NO TIME TO COOK BREAKFAST?

You can still follow this two-week meal plan—and the entire low-glycal way of eating—even if you don't have time to cook in the morning. Most workplaces have a break room with a fridge and microwave. As long as you have something you can grab from your fridge as you leave the house, you can enjoy a satisfying, healthful, low-glycal breakfast at work. Or, if you're a fan of a breakfast sandwich from the drive-thru, go ahead and order two but throw away the bread and eat only the egg, cheese and meat filling.

A TWO-WEEK LOW-GLYCAL MENU PLAN FOR STEP 1—KICK-START YOUR WEIGHT LOSS!

Note: All servings are "single," which are also defined in the recipes and in the companion Low-Glycal Diet app. Step 1 is the strictest part of the diet; you'll find more choices in Step 2 and Step 3.

DAY 1

Breakfast

- Egg/s—your way (fried, scrambled, poached)
- Bacon (2 slices) *or* sausage (2 links)
- Cantaloupe slices (¼ of the whole melon)
- Coffee or tea, unsweetened

Mid-morning snack

- Almonds, raw (¼ cup [36 g])
- Coffee or tea, unsweetened

Lunch

- Salade Niçoise (recipe on page 128)
- Coffee or tea, unsweetened

Mid-afternoon snack

- Apple (1)
- Coffee or tea, unsweetened

Dinner

- Chicken Tenders Provençale (recipe on page 139)
- Sautéed Swiss chard (1 cup [55 g], cooked)
- Salad of mixed baby greens, lightly dressed (1 cup [55 g] greens; 1½ teaspoons [7 g] dressing)
- Mineral water or wine

DAY 2

Breakfast

- All-bran cereal (½ cup [40 g])
- Almond milk, unsweetened (½ cup [120 ml])
- Blueberries (¼ cup [35 g])
- Coffee or tea, unsweetened

Mid-morning snack

- Celery sticks (3 stems) with Tzatziki Dip (recipe on page 189)
- Coffee or tea, unsweetened

Lunch

- Eggplant Salad (recipe on page 126)
- Tuna, packed in olive oil (one 5-ounce [140-g] can)
- Coffee or tea, unsweetened

Mid-morning snack

- Peanuts, dry-roasted (¼ cup [35 g])
- Coffee or tea, unsweetened

Dinner

- Grilled rib-eye steak
- Small Caesar Salad (recipe on page 169)
- Mineral water or wine

DAY 3

Breakfast

- Egg/s—your way (fried, scrambled, poached)
- Bacon (2 slices) or sausage (2 links)
- Grapefruit (½), unsweetened
- Coffee or tea, unsweetened

Mid-morning snack

- Cheese Sticks (recipe on page 185)
- Coffee or tea, unsweetened

Lunch

- Egg Salad, Ham and Lettuce Roll-Ups (recipe on page 125)
- Coffee or tea, unsweetened

Mid-afternoon snack

- Whole-grain bread (1 slice)
- Peanut butter, unsweetened (1 tablespoon [16 g])
- Coffee or tea, unsweetened

Dinner

- Parmesan Pork Chops (recipe on page 143)
- Roasted Brussels Sprouts (recipe on page 172)
- Salad of mixed greens, lightly dressed (1 cup [55 g] greens; 1½ teaspoons [7 g] dressing)
- Mineral water or wine

DAY 4

Breakfast

- Yogurt, whole milk, plain, unsweetened (1 cup [230 g])
- Strawberries, sliced (½ cup [85 g])
- Coffee or tea, unsweetened

Mid-morning snack

- Hard-boiled egg (1)
- Coffee or tea, unsweetened

Lunch

- Caprese Salad (recipe on page 120)
- Sardines, packed in olive oil (1 or 2 tins, 3.75 ounces [106 g] each)
- Coffee or tea, unsweetened

Mid-afternoon snack

- Banana (1)
- Coffee or tea, unsweetened

Dinner

- Herbed Whole-Roasted Chicken (recipe on page 141)
- Spinach, cooked; fresh or frozen (1 cup [180 g])
- Salad of mixed greens, lightly dressed (1 cup [55 g] greens; 1½ teaspoons [7 g] dressing)
- Mineral water or wine

DAY 5

Breakfast

- Oatmeal, steel-cut, with cinnamon (1 cup [80 g])
- Blueberries (½ cup [75 g]) *or* walnuts (¼ cup [30 g], chopped)
- Coffee or tea, unsweetened

Mid-morning snack

- Hummus (¼ cup [60 g]; recipe on page 187) on endive (4 leaves)
- Coffee or tea, unsweetened

Lunch

- Ham, cheese and lettuce roll-ups
- Grapes, red, sliced (½ cup [75 g])
- Coffee or tea, unsweetened

Mid-afternoon snack

- Walnuts, raw (¼ cup [30 g])
- Coffee or tea, unsweetened

Dinner

- Tuna Steak Mediterranean (recipe on page 165)
- Salad of mixed greens, lightly dressed (2 cups [110 g] greens; 2 teaspoons [10 g] dressing)
- Mineral water or wine

DAY 6

Breakfast
- Swiss Cheese Omelet (recipe on page 110)
- Bacon (2 slices)
- Avocado slices (½ an avocado)
- Coffee or tea, unsweetened

Mid-morning snack
- Whole-grain bread (1 slice)
- Peanut butter, unsweetened (1 tablespoon [16 g])
- Coffee or tea, unsweetened

Lunch
- Chicken Caesar Salad (no croutons)
- Coffee or tea, unsweetened

Mid-afternoon snack
- Pear (1)
- Coffee or tea, unsweetened

Dinner
- Grilled lamb shoulder chop (1)
- Green Bean Salad (recipe on page 178)
- Salad of mixed greens, lightly dressed (1 cup greens [55 g]; 1½ teaspoons [7 g] dressing)
- Mineral water or wine

DAY 7

Breakfast
- Egg, poached (1)
- Whole-grain bread, toasted (1 slice)
- Smoked salmon, thinly sliced (4 ounces [113 g])
- Grapefruit (½)
- Coffee or tea, unsweetened

Mid-morning snack

- Yogurt, whole milk, plain, unsweetened (1 cup [230 g])
- Fresh berries, unsweetened (raspberries, sliced strawberries or blueberries; ¼ cup [35 g])
- Coffee or tea, unsweetened

Lunch

- Cobb Salad (recipe on page 121)
- Coffee or tea, unsweetened

Mid-afternoon snack

- Apple (1)
- Almond butter, unsweetened (1 tablespoon [16 g])
- Coffee or tea, unsweetened

Dinner

- Fish Chowder (recipe on page 158)
- Salad of mixed greens, lightly dressed (1 cup greens [55 g]; 1½ teaspoons [7 g] dressing)
- Mineral water or wine

DAY 8

Breakfast

- Cheesy Baked Egg (one; recipe on page 111)
- Bacon (2 slices) *or* sausage (2 links)
- Grapefruit (½)
- Coffee or tea, unsweetened

Mid-morning snack

- Almonds, raw (¼ cup [36 g])
- Coffee or tea, unsweetened

Lunch

- Salmon Salad Lettuce Wraps (recipe on page 129)
- Coffee or tea, unsweetened

Mid-afternoon snack

- Fresh pineapple slices (3)
- Coffee or tea, unsweetened

Dinner

- Grilled Sirloin Steak (recipe on page 152)
- Spinach Salad with Bleu Cheese (recipe on page 168)
- Mineral water or wine

DAY 9

Breakfast

- Grape-Nuts cereal (½ cup [20 g])
- Almond milk, unsweetened (½ cup [120 ml])
- Blueberries (¼ cup [35 g])
- Coffee or tea, unsweetened

Mid-morning snack

- Hard-boiled egg (1)
- Coffee or tea, unsweetened

Lunch

- Tarragon Chicken Salad (recipe on page 131)
- Coffee or tea, unsweetened

Mid-afternoon snack

- Cottage cheese (½ cup [115 g])
- Peanuts, dry-roasted (¼ cup [35 g])
- Coffee or tea, unsweetened

Dinner

- Baked Cod Provençale (recipe on page 157)
- Garlic Green Beans (recipe on page 177)
- Salad of mixed greens, lightly dressed (1 cup greens [55 g]; 1½ teaspoons [7 g] dressing)
- Mineral water or wine

DAY 10

Breakfast

- Egg/s—your way (fried, scrambled, poached)
- Bacon (2 slices) *or* sausage (2 links)
- Grapefruit (½)
- Coffee or tea, unsweetened

Mid-morning snack

- Savory Cheese Spread (2 tablespoons [30 g]; recipe on page 186) on endive (4 leaves)
- Coffee or tea, unsweetened

Lunch

- Curried Shrimp Salad (recipe on page 124)
- Coffee or tea, unsweetened

Mid-afternoon snack

- Fruit salad of orange, grapefruit and strawberries, unsweetened (1 cup [150 g])
- Coffee or tea, unsweetened

Dinner

- Parmesan Chicken Breasts (recipe on page 142)
- Cauliflower Casserole (recipe on page 176)
- Salad of mixed greens, lightly dressed (1 cup greens [55 g]; 1½ teaspoons [7 g] dressing)
- Mineral water or wine

DAY 11

Breakfast

- Yogurt, whole milk, plain, unsweetened (1 cup [230 g])
- Blueberries or blackberries (½ cup [75 g])
- Coffee or tea, unsweetened

Mid-morning snack

- Cheese Sticks (recipe on page 185)
- Coffee or tea, unsweetened

Lunch

- Egg Salad with Chopped Ham (recipe on page 125)
- Coffee or tea, unsweetened

Mid-afternoon snack

- Endive with Marseille-Style Sardine Spread (recipe on page 188)
- Coffee or tea, unsweetened

Dinner

- Mustard Glazed Pork (recipe on page 145)
- Red Cabbage with Caraway Seeds (recipe on page 174)
- Carrots, steamed; fresh or frozen (½ cup [60 g])
- Mineral water or wine

DAY 12

Breakfast

- Cheese Omelet (recipe on page 110)
- Bacon (2 slices) *or* sausage (2 links)
- Honeydew melon (¼ of the melon)
- Coffee or tea, unsweetened

Mid-morning snack

- Red grapes, sliced (1 cup [150 g])
- Coffee or tea, unsweetened

Lunch

- Tomato soup
- Cheese Sticks (recipe on page 185)
- Coffee or tea, unsweetened

Mid-afternoon snack

- Whole-grain bread (1 slice)
- Peanut butter, unsweetened (1 tablespoon [16 g])
- Coffee or tea, unsweetened

Dinner

- Baked Flounder (recipe on page 135)
- Asparagus, steamed; fresh or frozen (6–8 spears)
- Salad of mixed greens, lightly dressed (1 cup [55 g] greens; 1½ teaspoons [7 g] dressing)
- Mineral water or wine

DAY 13

Breakfast

- Oatmeal, steel-cut, with cinnamon (1 cup [80 g]), mixed with chopped apple
- Chopped apple (1)
- Coffee or tea, unsweetened

Mid-morning snack

- Whole-grain bread (1 slice)
- Almond butter, unsweetened (1 tablespoon [16 g])
- Coffee or tea, unsweetened

Lunch

- Turkey salad (see Tarragon Chicken Salad recipe on page 131)
- Coffee or tea, unsweetened

Mid-afternoon snack

- Almonds, raw (¼ cup [36 g])
- Coffee or tea, unsweetened

Dinner

- Baked Salmon Steak (recipe on page 135)
- Broccoli, roasted (1 cup [70 g]) tossed with 1 teaspoon sesame oil
- Salad of mixed greens, lightly dressed (1 cup [55 g] greens; 1½ teaspoons [7 g] dressing)
- Mineral water or wine

DAY 14

Breakfast

- Egg/s—your way (fried, scrambled, poached)
- Broiled tomato (one; recipe on page 117)
- Cantaloupe (¼ of the melon)
- Coffee or tea, unsweetened

Mid-morning snack

- Cheese Sticks (recipe on page 185)
- Coffee or tea, unsweetened

Lunch

- Crabmeat and Avocado Salad (recipe on page 123)
- Coffee or tea, unsweetened

Mid-afternoon snack

- Celery (3 stems)
- Goat cheese (2 tablespoons [28 g])
- Coffee or tea, unsweetened

Dinner

- Prime rib roast
- Arugula, Walnut and Goat Cheese Salad
- Mineral water or wine

CHAPTER 5

STEP 2: REACH YOUR IDEAL WEIGHT—WITH THE MODIFIED MEAL PLAN

Good news! You've completed Step 1 and kick-started your weight loss. You feel lighter, more energetic, and can already see the changes in your body. Now, you're ready for the second phase of the Low-Glycal Diet: Step 2. And, guess what? This part of the diet is even easier than the first!

MORE EFFORTLESS WEIGHT LOSS

In Step 2, you will be adding one medium-glycal meal a day (coded "yellow" in the companion app) to your menus, and you can even have one high-glycal meal ("red") per week. You will continue to lose weight and fat during Step 2, without experiencing the fatigue and hunger common to so many diet plans. And now, you can start adding back some of the foods you may have been missing. You'll find ideas for that in the meal plan suggestions that follow.

You will stay on this part of the plan until you have reached your ideal weight. And because you can mix-and-match this 14-day meal plan indefinitely with menus from Step 1, the variety and flexibility of Step 2 will keep you motivated and comfortable as you keep dropping the pounds. Remember, too, that you can make your own meal plans of low- and medium-glycal dishes by looking through the recipes in Chapter 7, where all the recipes are coded as green, yellow or red.

You are going to find that the good habits you developed during Step 1 will make following Step 2 a snap. As you enjoy even more food choices and meal options during this part of the diet, you will continue to lose fat while you maintain or increase lean body mass. You will also continue to slow the aging process because you'll avoid spikes in your blood sugar with your new way of eating.

After two weeks of low-glycal eating during Step 1, you'll notice that you have not only lost weight but also some of your old cravings, particularly for sweets. That's one of the benefits of this diet. But even though your cravings have changed, it's good to know that during Step 2 you will be able to enjoy certain items that you may have been missing. That's right—you can say *yes* to that invitation to go out for burgers and fries with your co-workers on Friday (that will be your red meal for the week). And the next week, you can do it again. Or, maybe you'd rather revisit your tradition of a pasta dinner on Wednesdays. Fine, that's your red meal for the week. In other words, now that you can have one high-glycal meal a week, it's easier than ever to stick with the low-glycal diet.

Now, during Step 2, you'll be replacing one green (low-glycal) meal a day with a yellow (medium-glycal) meal. Every day. This feature is why the Low-Glycal Diet is truly easy to stick with. The expanded food choices in Step 2 mean you'll enjoy even greater variety in your meals, you won't be hungry and you will continue to lose weight and fat without feeling like you are in a state of deprivation. So when you feel you've simply got to have that lasagna, go ahead—it's a red (high-glycal) meal but you'll still be following the diet!

The Low-Glycal Diet takes into account the special occasions of real life. Your parent's anniversary party, your nephew's wedding, your boss's retirement dinner—go ahead, enjoy yourself. These examples are all red (high-glycal) meal occasions but you can make them work during Step 2 by creating a meal plan each week that accounts for *your* real life.

During Step 2, you just need to maintain the right balance of mostly "green" meals, some "yellow," and a little "red" until you've reached your ideal weight. The meal plan that follows has 14 days' worth of suggestions. Between that and the recipes in Chapter 7, you will find this phase of the diet easy. And, you'll continue to lose weight and regain energy.

HOW TO DRESS A SALAD

Are you in the habit of pouring on a *lot* more salad dressing than needed, leaving a large puddle of dressing at the bottom of your salad bowl (wasting it), or adding significantly to the calorie load of what you probably consider a low-cal side dish? Now that you are tuned-in to more thoughtful shopping, food prep and meal planning with the Low-Glycal Diet, use your new awareness when you dress a salad. For a small side-salad (a cup of packed torn or chopped lettuce or mixed small-leaf lettuces) all you need is a teaspoon and a half of salad dressing or a drizzle of good olive oil and a sprinkle of vinegar. Add a pinch of salt and freshly ground pepper and toss well. Chef's tip: use a much larger bowl than needed to toss the greens, which will allow them to be evenly coated with the salad dressing; then, transfer to a small salad plate.

This chapter includes a 2-week menu plan for three meals a day (plus mid-morning and mid-afternoon snacks) that allows for one medium-glycal meal a day ("yellow"), and one high-glycal meal a week ("red"); all the other meals or snacks are low-glycal ("green"). The meal plan that follows is a *suggestion*; you can vary the dishes to suit your schedule, tastes and budget, just as you did with the 14-day meal plan for Step 1 of the diet. Check out the recipes again or consult the companion app and use the templates in Chapter 9 to create a week-by-week meal plan that's perfect for you. For example, if the best day of the week for you to have that red meal is Thursday, plan for it. As long as you follow the design of Step 2—no more than one yellow meal a day and no more than one red meal a week—you'll be fine.

You will be following Step 2 until you reach your desired weight. By combining the meal plans in this chapter and the 14-day plan included in Chapter 3, you will have 28 days' worth of suggestions for breakfasts, lunches, dinners and snacks to work with. And, you can peruse the recipes in Chapter 7 for dishes that may not have appeared yet. In other words, you can truly mix and match menus indefinitely during Step 2 of the low-glycal diet. With the help of the free Low-Glycal Diet companion app, you can create your own meals plans to suit your lifestyle, schedule and pocketbook.

The "one medium-glycal meal a day" rule in Step 2 allows you to decide when you want that treat; it can be at breakfast, lunch or dinner. The same is true with the "one red meal a week" rule during Step 2. If you've been craving waffles,

IS THE GLYCAL A CHAMELEON?

Keep in mind that what may be a red or yellow meal in the evening is often a yellow or green meal at lunch. That information is frequently noted in the recipes for main course dishes but you can also determine the color change in a meal, which is based on the time of day that you eat it, by consulting the free companion app. This chameleon-like quality of the meals actually means you have more flexibility with the Low-Glycal Diet than any other diet.

your red meal will probably be a weekend brunch; if you've been craving mashed potatoes with steak, that red meal will probably be a dinner. The flexibility of Step 2 in the Low-Glycal Diet means you can make the plan work for you!

Remember: During Step 2 you will still follow the two-hours-between-meals-and-snacks rule and avoid eating after 8:00 p.m.

"This is your world. Shape it or someone else will." —Gary Lew

A successful life requires planning. Healthful meals do, too! Now that you've reached Step 2 in the Low-Glycal Diet, be sure to keep planning your meals for the week ahead. That way, you'll know when your red (high-glycal) meal is coming up and you can look forward to it.

You'll also figure out where you want your yellow (medium-glycal) meals to show up throughout the week; you may not want to change your standard low-glycal breakfast of a scrambled egg and sausage, or your go-to low-glycal dinner of a grilled chop, a green vegetable and small salad. If that's you, you can now enjoy a medium-glycal lunch every day. Terrific! Put it in writing, in your personal meal plan. See the template in Chapter 9.

ADVANCING TO STEP 2 THE SMART WAY

Smart Tip: During Step 2, you'll probably find that getting a single serving of that yellow or red meal "to-go" from the prepared foods counter at your market is a good move. (Do you really want a whole pan of homemade lasagna staring at you every time you open the fridge?) Or, if you want a scone with strawberry jam as a treat, put it on your meal plan to meet a friend at your favorite bakery café for a cup of coffee. You'll enjoy a red treat, and the chance to catch up with a friend.

You *will* find recipes in this book for medium-glycal and high-glycal meals, but they are mostly for items that contain low-glycal staples or that yield excellent leftover low-glycal lunches.

A TWO-WEEK MEAL PLAN FOR STEP 2 IN THE LOW-GLYCAL DIET

DAY 1

Breakfast

- All-bran cereal (½ cup [40 g])
- Almond milk, unsweetened (½ cup [120 ml])
- Blueberries (¼ cup [35 g])
- Coffee or tea, unsweetened

Mid-morning snack

- Hard-boiled egg (1)
- Coffee or tea, unsweetened

Lunch (yellow meal)

- Tuna salad sandwich (½ cup [112 g] tuna salad, lettuce, in a ½ piece pita bread)
- Coffee or tea, unsweetened

Mid-afternoon snack

- Bagel (½), toasted (wrap and store the other half in the fridge or freezer)
- Cream cheese (1 tablespoon [15 g])
- Coffee or tea, unsweetened

Dinner

- Chicken with White Wine (recipe on page 140)
- Broccoli, steamed; fresh or frozen (1 cup [70 g])
- Salad of mixed greens, lightly dressed (1 cup [55 g] greens; 1½ teaspoons [7 g] dressing)
- Mineral water or wine

DAY 2

Breakfast (yellow meal)

- Sausage Frittata (recipe on page 116)
- Whole-grain toast (1 piece)
- Grapefruit, unsweetened (½)
- Coffee or tea, unsweetened

Mid-morning snack

- Almonds, raw (¼ cup [36 g])
- Coffee or tea, unsweetened

Lunch

- Ham, cheese and lettuce roll-ups
- Coffee or tea, unsweetened

Mid-afternoon snack

- Carrots (3 whole) cut into sticks
- Ranch-style dressing (2 tablespoons [30 g]), for dipping
- Coffee or tea, unsweetened

Dinner

- Baked Haddock (recipe on page 135)
- Vegetable Gratin (recipe on page 182)
- Salad of mixed greens, lightly dressed (1 cup [55 g] greens; 1½ teaspoons [7 g] dressing)
- Mineral water or wine

DAY 3

Breakfast

- Oatmeal, steel-cut, with cinnamon (1 cup [80 g])
- Banana (½, save the other half for morning snack)
- Coffee or tea, unsweetened

Mid-morning snack

- Banana (½)
- Peanut butter, unsweetened (1 tablespoon [16 g])
- Coffee or tea, unsweetened

Lunch

- Asian Chicken Salad (recipe on page 119)
- Coffee or tea, unsweetened

Mid-afternoon snack (yellow snack)

- Corn muffin
- Coffee or tea, unsweetened

Dinner

- Grilled lamb chop (1 shoulder chop)
- Roasted Cauliflower with Capers (recipe on page 175)
- Salad of mixed greens, lightly dressed (1 cup [55 g] greens; 1½ teaspoons [7 g] dressing)
- Mineral water or wine

DAY 4

Breakfast

- Egg/s—your way (fried, scrambled, poached)
- Bacon (2 slices) *or* sausage (2 links)
- Clementine (1)
- Coffee or tea, unsweetened

Mid-morning snack

- Celery (3 stems)
- Peanut butter, unsweetened (1 tablespoon [16 g])
- Coffee or tea, unsweetened

Lunch (yellow meal)

- Steak and Bean Burrito (recipe on page 130)
- Coffee or tea, unsweetened

Mid-afternoon snack

- Cheese Sticks (recipe on page 185)
- Coffee or tea, unsweetened

Dinner

- Crustless Salmon Quiche (recipe on page 162)
- Broccoli, steamed; fresh or frozen (1 cup [70 g])
- Salad of mixed greens, lightly dressed (1 cup [55 g] greens; 1½ teaspoons [7 g] dressing)
- Mineral water or wine

DAY 5

Breakfast (yellow meal)

- Egg, fried over-easy (1)
- Toast (2 slices, buttered with ½ tablespoon [7 g] butter)
- Fruit salad
- Coffee or tea, unsweetened

Mid-morning snack

- Hummus (¼ cup [60 g]; recipe on page 187) on endive (4 pieces)
- Coffee or tea, unsweetened

Lunch

- Clam Chowder (recipe on page 122)
- Apple (1)
- Coffee or tea, unsweetened

Mid-afternoon snack

- Walnuts, raw (¼ cup [25 g])
- Coffee or tea, unsweetened

Dinner

- Baked country-style ham with mustard glaze
- Asparagus, steamed; fresh or frozen (6 stalks)
- Salad of mixed greens, lightly dressed (1 cup [55 g] greens; 1½ teaspoons [7 g] dressing)
- Mineral water or wine

DAY 6

Breakfast

- Toasted multi-grain bread (1 slice) with cream cheese (1 tablespoon [15 g]) and smoked salmon (2 slices)
- Cantaloupe (¼ of a whole melon)
- Coffee or tea, unsweetened

Mid-morning snack

- Hard-boiled egg (1)
- Coffee or tea, unsweetened

Lunch (yellow meal)

- Tomato soup (1 cup [235 ml]) with ¼ cup [30 g] croutons)
- Ham, cheese and lettuce roll-ups
- Coffee or tea, unsweetened

Mid-afternoon snack

- Peanuts, dry roasted (¼ cup [35 g])
- Coffee or tea, unsweetened

Dinner

- Garlic Shrimp (recipe on page 164)
- Green Bean Salad (recipe on page 178)
- Salad of mixed greens, lightly dressed (1 cup [55 g] greens; 1½ teaspoons [7 g] dressing)
- Mineral water or wine

DAY 7

Breakfast

- Asparagus Frittata (recipe on page 115)
- Grapefruit (½)
- Coffee or tea, unsweetened

Mid-morning snack

- Yogurt, plain unsweetened (1 cup [230 g])
- Fresh berries, unsweetened (¼ cup [35 g] raspberries, sliced strawberries or blueberries)
- Coffee or tea, unsweetened

Lunch (red meal)

- Lasagna (1 serving)
- Garlic bread
- Tossed salad
- Coffee or tea, unsweetened

Mid-afternoon snack

- Whole-grain bread (1 slice)
- Almond butter, unsweetened (1 tablespoon [16 g])
- Coffee or tea, unsweetened

Dinner

- Crabmeat Salad Plate (recipe on page 123)
- Mineral water or wine

DAY 8

Breakfast

- Oatmeal, steel-cut, with cinnamon (1 cup [80 g])
- Blackberries (½ cup [75 g])
- Coffee or tea, unsweetened

Mid-morning snack

- Hard-boiled egg (1)
- Coffee or tea, unsweetened

Lunch

- Vegetable Soup (recipe on page 133)
- Coffee or tea, unsweetened

Mid-afternoon snack (yellow snack)

- Bran muffin
- Coffee or tea, unsweetened

Dinner

- Flank Steak (recipe on page 150)
- Spinach, steamed; fresh or frozen (1 cup [180 g])
- Small Caesar Salad (recipe on page 169)
- Mineral water or wine

DAY 9

Breakfast

- Cheddar Cheese Omelet (recipe on page 110)
- Bacon (2 pieces)
- Coffee or tea, unsweetened

Mid-morning snack

- Green grapes (1 cup [150 g])
- Coffee or tea, unsweetened

Lunch (yellow meal)

- Steak and Bean Burrito (recipe on page 130)
- Coffee or tea, unsweetened

Mid-afternoon snack

- Peanuts, dry roasted (¼ cup [35 g])
- Coffee or tea, unsweetened

Dinner

- Seared Scallops with Summer Corn and Tomatoes (recipe on page 117)
- Mineral water or wine

DAY 10

Breakfast

- Egg, scrambled (1)
- Broiled Tomato (recipe on page 117)
- Coffee or tea, unsweetened

Mid-morning snack

- Celery, 3 stems
- Savory Cheese Spread (2 tablespoons [28 g]; recipe on page 186)
- Coffee or tea, unsweetened

Lunch (yellow meal)

- Lamb Burger (recipe on page 149)
- Coffee or tea, unsweetened

Mid-afternoon snack

- Apple (1)
- Coffee or tea, unsweetened

Dinner

- Tarragon Chicken Salad (recipe on page 131)
- Mineral water or wine

DAY 11

Breakfast (yellow meal)

- French toast topped with sliced strawberries
- Coffee or tea, unsweetened

Mid-morning snack

- Cheese Sticks (recipe on page 185)
- Coffee or tea, unsweetened

Lunch

- Zucchini Frittata (recipe on page 115)
- Cherry tomatoes, halved (½ cup [75 g]), with Basic Salad Dressing (recipe on page 183)
- Coffee or tea, unsweetened

Mid-afternoon snack

- Walnuts, raw (¼ cup [30 g])
- Coffee or tea, unsweetened

Dinner

- Baked Flounder (recipe on page 135)
- Broccoli, steamed; fresh or frozen (1 cup [70 g])
- Small Caesar Salad (recipe on page 169)
- Mineral water or wine

DAY 12

Breakfast

- Grape-Nuts cereal (½ cup [40 g])
- Almond milk, unsweetened (½ cup 120 ml])
- Blueberries (¼ cup [35 g])
- Coffee or tea, unsweetened

Mid-morning snack

- Hard-boiled egg (1)
- Coffee or tea, unsweetened

Lunch (yellow meal)

- Curried Shrimp Salad (recipe on page 124)
- Fruit sorbet (½ cup [75 g])
- Coffee or tea, unsweetened

Mid-afternoon snack

- Whole-grain bread (1 slice)
- Peanut butter, unsweetened (1 tablespoon [16 g])
- Coffee or tea, unsweetened

Dinner

- Parmesan and Honey Roast Pork Tenderloin (recipe on page 146)
- Savory Savoy Cabbage (recipe on page 172)
- Salad of mixed greens, lightly dressed (1 cup [55 g] greens; 1½ teaspoons [7 g] dressing)
- Mineral water or wine

DAY 13

Breakfast

- Eggs Florentine (recipe on page 112)
- Grapefruit (½)
- Coffee or tea, unsweetened

Mid-morning snack

- Red grapes (1 cup [150 g])
- Coffee or tea, unsweetened

Lunch (yellow meal)

- BLT sandwich, open faced
- Coffee or tea, unsweetened

Mid-afternoon snack

- Edamame (¼ cup [40 g])
- Coffee or tea, unsweetened

Dinner

- Oyster Spinach Salad (recipe on page 161)
- Mineral water or wine

DAY 14

Breakfast

- Egg, scrambled (1)
- Bacon (2 pieces)
- Cantaloupe slices (¼ of whole melon)
- Coffee or tea, unsweetened

Mid-morning snack

- Cheese Sticks (recipe on page 185)
- Coffee or tea, unsweetened

Lunch

- Lobster Salad (recipe on page 127)
- Coffee or tea, unsweetened

Mid-afternoon snack

- Apple (1)
- Coffee or tea, unsweetened

Dinner (red meal)

- Whole Roasted Sirloin (recipe on page 154)
- Spinach Soufflé (recipe on page 168)
- Red-skin potatoes, boiled, skin left on
- Fennel, Endive and Orange Salad (recipe on page 167)
- Mineral water or wine

CHAPTER 6

STEP 3: MAINTENANCE— KEEP THE WEIGHT OFF LONG TERM

Congratulations—you have achieved your weight-loss goal and reached your ideal weight! And, you have also slowed down the aging process, greatly improving your overall health. The differences are apparent in ways you can clearly see and feel, as well as at the cellular level, too. While you can't look in the mirror and see what's going on in your organs and vascular system, the rejuvenation taking place there is significant and has a tremendous effect on your quality of life—now, and in the years to come.

Once you have reached your weight-loss goal, you are finished with Step 2 of the Low-Glycal Diet plan and are ready to move on to Step 3, the maintenance phase of the diet. This is a plan you can live with for life.

During this phase, you will continue eating much the same way as you have become accustomed to in Step 2: For six days a week you will have two green (low-glycal) meals and one yellow (medium-glycal) meal a day *plus* all the green (low-glycal) snacks you want—as long as meals and snacks are separated by two hours, and as long as you stop eating by eight o'clock at night.

Okay, you're thinking, *but there are seven days in a week. What's different on the seventh day?*

In Step 3, one day a week—and this is a *big* difference—you are allowed to eat whatever you want, whenever you want. I call this the "cheat" day, and you get one a week, *every week*, forever! On the "cheat" day, you can eat all the red (high-glycal) meals you want, and you can disregard the two-hour rule, too. This part of the diet means the maintenance plan is extremely easy to stick with.

Now, just because Step 3 includes a cheat day once a week, you shouldn't feel obligated to indulge in junk food. By now, you have probably lost all your old cravings and don't even have a desire for some of the items you used to eat. And that's a good thing! Certainly, I urge you to keep high-fructose corn syrup out of your diet forever, and I encourage you to stay mindful of the difference between processed grains and whole grains. The change in restrictions on red (high-glycal) meals simply allows you even more flexibility and fun—a high-glycal dinner at your favorite restaurant, an extravagant brunch party for friends, a pull-out-all-the-stops family dinner or a casual clam-shack meal of clam fritters,

WEIGHT MAINTENANCE GUIDELINES

In Step 3 you are maintaining your ideal weight. Every week, you will follow a seven-day plan that looks like this:

Six days a week, you will be eating:

• Two green (low-glycal) meals and one yellow (medium-glycal) meal a day

• Two green (low-glycal) snacks, one mid-morning and one mid-afternoon (or more if your schedule allows)

One day a week, you will be eating:

• Whatever you want! Red (high-glycal) meals and snacks, without regard to the two-hour rule!

chowder, French fries and ice cream—virtually whatever works for you can be part of Step 3 and your ongoing weight maintenance. My guess, however, is that your tastes and sensibilities have changed to the degree that even on the cheat day you'll be making smarter choices than before you began the Low-Glycal Diet.

MAINTAINING YOUR IDEAL WEIGHT THE SMART WAY

Remember the "smart tip" for Step 2 that recommended you visit the prepared foods counter at your market to purchase a single serving of whatever red (or even yellow) meal might be on your week's plan? That's still a good idea. Your fridge, freezer and cupboards should be stocked with everything you need for green (low-glycal) eating so that you continue to follow the Low-Glycal Diet with ease and success.

This chapter gives you another 14-day meal plan. This one contains green, yellow and red meals that fit the weight maintenance phase of the Low-Glycal Diet. This meal plan and all the suggestions in the meal plans contained in Chapter 4 and Chapter 5 gives you literally dozens of options to mix and match menus to suit your tastes, schedule and budget while you continue to enjoy the life-long benefits of the Low-Glycal Diet.

TIMING IS EVERYTHING

Even during Step 3, the long-term maintenance phase of the Low-Glycal Diet,
timing counts. Remember to separate all meals and snacks by two hours, and do
not eat after eight o'clock at night EXCEPT one day a week when anything goes!
Call it your "cheat day," when you can eat all the red meals or snacks you want,
and without regard to the two-hour rule.

A PLAN YOU CAN LIVE WITH

The Low-Glycal Diet really is a plan you can stick with for life—and you'll want
to because you'll feel and look so good, and because the meal plan is realistic.
Healthful, and delicious, the menus that follow will round out your new way of
eating. Enjoy!

A TWO-WEEK MENU PLAN FOR STEP 3 IN THE LOW-GLYCAL DIET

DAY 1

Breakfast

- Egg/s—your way (fried, scrambled, poached)
- Bacon (2 slices) *or* sausage (2 links)
- Grapefruit (½) unsweetened
- Coffee or tea, unsweetened

Mid-morning snack

- Bagel (½), toasted (wrap and store the other half in the fridge or freezer)
- Cream cheese (1 tablespoon [15 g])
- Coffee or tea, unsweetened

Lunch (yellow meal)

- Open-face turkey-melt sandwich
- Coffee or tea, unsweetened

Mid-afternoon snack

- Peanuts, dry-roasted (¼ cup [35 g])
- Coffee or tea, unsweetened

Dinner

- Baked Salmon Filet (recipe on page 135)
- Peas, steamed; fresh or frozen (½ cup [85 g])
- Salad of mixed greens, lightly dressed (1 cup [55 g] greens; 1½ teaspoons [7 g] dressing)
- Mineral water or wine

DAY 2

Breakfast

- Oatmeal, steel-cut, with cinnamon (1 cup [80 g])
- Blueberries (½ cup [75 g])
- Coffee or tea, unsweetened

Mid-morning snack

- Hard-boiled egg (1)
- Coffee or tea, unsweetened

Lunch (yellow meal)

- Tuna Salad Roll-Ups (recipe on page 132)
- Potato chips (a 1-ounce [28-g] bag])
- Coffee or tea, unsweetened

Mid-afternoon snack

- Pear (1)
- Coffee or tea, unsweetened

Dinner

- Baked Pork Spare Ribs (recipe on page 144)
- Cole slaw (½ cup [75 g]; be sure it has no sugar in it)
- Mineral water or wine

DAY 3

Breakfast

- Cheese Omelet (recipe on page 110)
- Bacon (2 slices) *or* sausage (2 links)
- Honeydew melon slices (¼ of the whole melon)
- Coffee or tea, unsweetened

Mid-morning snack

- Apple (1)
- Coffee or tea, unsweetened

Lunch

- Asian Chicken Salad (recipe on page 119)
- Coffee or tea, unsweetened

Mid-afternoon snack

- Bagel (½) toasted
- Cottage cheese (½ cup [115 g])
- Coffee or tea, unsweetened

Dinner (yellow meal)

- Grilled Swordfish Steak (recipe on page 135)
- Herbed Green Beans (recipe on page 180)
- Corn on the cob (1 ear)
- Mineral water or wine

DAY 4

Breakfast

- Grape-Nuts cereal (½ cup [40 g])
- Almond milk, unsweetened (½ cup [120 ml])
- Blueberries (¼ cup [35 g])
- Coffee or tea, unsweetened

Mid-morning snack

- Cheese Sticks (recipe on page 185)
- Coffee or tea, unsweetened

Lunch (yellow meal)

- Black bean burrito (flour tortilla, black beans, guacamole, cheese, salsa)
- Coffee or tea, unsweetened

Mid-afternoon snack

- Almonds, raw (¼ cup [36 g])
- Coffee or tea, unsweetened

Dinner

- Wine-Braised Short Ribs (recipe on page 153)
- Broccoli, steamed; fresh or frozen (1 cup [70 g])
- Salad of mixed greens, lightly dressed (1 cup [55 g] greens; 1½ teaspoons [7 g] dressing)
- Mineral water or wine

DAY 5

Breakfast

- Egg/s—your way (fried, scrambled, poached)
- Bacon (2 slices) *or* sausage (2 links)
- Grapefruit (½), unsweetened
- Coffee or tea, unsweetened

Mid-morning snack

- Hummus (¼ cup [60 g]; recipe on page 187) on endive (4 leaves)
- Coffee or tea, unsweetened

Lunch (yellow meal)

- Pasta salad (1 cup [275 g])
- Sardines (1 tin, 3.75 ounces [106 g])
- Coffee or tea, unsweetened

Mid-afternoon snack

- Cashews, raw (¼ cup [35 g])
- Coffee or tea, unsweetened

Dinner

- Beef Provençale Style (recipe on page 148)
- Salad of mixed greens, lightly dressed (1 cup [55 g] greens; 1½ teaspoons [7 g] dressing)
- Mineral water or wine

DAY 6

Breakfast

- Multi-grain bread (1 slice) with cream cheese (1 tablespoon [15 g]) and smoked salmon (2 slices)
- Cantaloupe slices (¼ of a whole melon)
- Coffee or tea, unsweetened

Mid-morning snack

- Edamame (¼ cup [40 g])
- Coffee or tea, unsweetened

Lunch

- Egg salad on bed of salad greens
- Cherry tomatoes, halved (½ cup [75 g])
- Coffee or tea, unsweetened

Mid-afternoon snack

- Cheese Sticks (recipe on page 185)
- Coffee or tea, unsweetened

Dinner (yellow meal)

- Veal Cutlets with Basil (recipe on page 156)
- Carrots steamed, fresh or frozen (½ cup [65 g])
- Salad of mixed greens, lightly dressed (1 cup [55 g] greens; 1½ teaspoons [7 g] dressing)
- Mineral water or wine

DAY 7

Breakfast (red meal)

- Eggs Benedict (recipe on page 113)
- Parmesan Potatoes (recipe on page 181)
- Fruit salad
- Coffee or tea, unsweetened

Mid-morning snack (red snack)

- Sticky-top cinnamon bun
- Coffee or tea, unsweetened

Lunch (red meal)

- Open-face tuna melt sandwich
- Potato chips
- Coffee or tea, unsweetened

Mid-afternoon snack (red snack)

- Guacamole (recipe on page 170)
- Corn chips
- Coffee or tea, unsweetened

Dinner (red meal)

- Leeks, Pea & Mushrooms with Grilled Italian Sausage over Pasta (recipe on page 147)
- Italian bread
- Salad of mixed greens, lightly dressed
- Mineral water or wine

DAY 8

Breakfast

- Oatmeal, steel-cut, with cinnamon (1 cup [80 g])
- Peach, sliced (1)
- Coffee or tea, unsweetened

Mid-morning snack

- Apple (1)
- Coffee or tea, unsweetened

Lunch

- Zucchini Frittata (recipe on page 114)
- Broiled Tomato (recipe on page 117)
- Coffee or tea, unsweetened

Mid-afternoon snack

- Almonds, raw (¼ cup [35 g])
- Coffee or tea, unsweetened

Dinner (yellow meal)

- Baked Cod (recipe on page 135)
- Brown rice (½ cup [95 g] cooked rice)
- Small Caesar Salad (recipe on page 169)
- Mineral water

DAY 9

Breakfast

- Mushroom Omelet (recipe on page 110)
- Bacon (2 pieces)
- Coffee or tea, unsweetened

Mid-morning snack

- Green grapes (1 cup [150 g])
- Coffee or tea, unsweetened

Lunch (yellow meal)

- Seafood Chowder (recipe on page 159)
- Sourdough bread (1 slice or small roll)
- Coffee or tea, unsweetened

Mid-afternoon snack

- Cheese Sticks (recipe on page 185)
- Coffee or tea, unsweetened

Dinner

- Pot Roast (recipe on page 155)
- Brussels Sprouts with Bacon (recipe on page 171)
- Salad of mixed greens, lightly dressed (1 cup [55 g] greens; 1½ teaspoons [7 g] dressing)
- Mineral water or wine

DAY 10

Breakfast

- Egg/s—your way (fried, scrambled, poached)
- Bacon (2 slices) *or* sausage (2 links)
- Grapefruit (½), unsweetened
- Coffee or tea, unsweetened

Mid-morning snack

- Apple (1)
- Coffee or tea, unsweetened

Lunch (yellow meal)

- Black bean burrito (flour tortilla, black beans, guacamole, cheese, salsa)
- Coffee or tea, unsweetened

Mid-afternoon snack

- Celery (3 stems)
- Savory Cheese Spread (2 tablespoons [28 g]; recipe on page 186)
- Coffee or tea, unsweetened

Dinner

- Sautéed scallops
- Swiss chard, sautéed (1 cup [55 g])
- Salad of mixed greens, lightly dressed (1 cup [55 g] greens; 1½ teaspoons [7 g] dressing)
- Mineral water or wine

DAY 11

Breakfast (yellow meal)

- Bagel (½), toasted
- Peanut butter, unsweetened (1 tablespoon [16 g])
- Coffee or tea, unsweetened

Mid-morning snack

- Cheese Sticks (recipe on page 185)
- Coffee or tea, unsweetened

Lunch

- Lobster Salad (recipe on page 127)
- Coffee or tea, unsweetened

Mid-afternoon snack

- Walnuts, raw (¼ cup [35 g])
- Coffee or tea, unsweetened

Dinner

- Zucchini Frittata (recipe on page 115)
- Salad of mixed greens, lightly dressed (1 cup [55 g] greens; 1½ teaspoons [7 g] dressing)
- Mineral water or wine

DAY 12

Breakfast

- Yogurt, whole milk, plain, unsweetened (1 cup [230 g])
- Strawberries, sliced, unsweetened (½ cup [75 g])
- Coffee or tea, unsweetened

Mid-morning snack

- Hard-boiled egg (1)
- Coffee or tea, unsweetened

Lunch (yellow meal)

- Chicken Caesar wrap
- Coffee or tea, unsweetened

Mid-afternoon snack

- Whole-grain bread (1 slice)
- Almond butter, unsweetened (1 tablespoon [15 g])
- Coffee or tea, unsweetened

Dinner

- Hamburger, grilled (8 ounces [225 g])
- Small Caesar Salad (recipe on page 169)
- Spinach (fresh or frozen), steamed (1 cup [180 g])
- Mineral water or wine

DAY 13

Breakfast

- Egg, poached (1)
- Tomato slices, grilled (2)
- Bacon (2 slices)
- Coffee or tea, unsweetened

Mid-morning snack

- Orange (1)
- Coffee or tea, unsweetened

Lunch (yellow meal)

- Open-faced turkey, bacon, lettuce and tomato sandwich (on 1 piece of bread)
- Coffee or tea, unsweetened

Mid-afternoon snack

- Cheese Sticks (recipe on page 185)
- Coffee or tea, unsweetened

Dinner

- Crab Cakes (recipe on page 160)
- Herbed Green Beans (recipe on page 180)
- Salad of mixed greens, lightly dressed (1 cup [55 g] greens; 1½ teaspoons [7 g] dressing)
- Mineral water or wine

DAY 14

Breakfast (red meal)

- Blueberry pancakes with maple syrup
- Sausage (2 links)
- Cantaloupe (¼ of a whole melon)
- Coffee or tea, unsweetened

Mid-morning snack (red snack)

- Buttered popcorn
- Coffee or tea, unsweetened

Lunch (red meal)

- Grilled ham and cheese sandwich with potato chips and pickles
- Coffee or tea, unsweetened

Mid-afternoon snack (red snack)

- Hummus (recipe on page 187) with pita chips
- Coffee or tea, unsweetened

Dinner (red meal)

- Rack of lamb
- Spinach Soufflé (recipe on page 112)
- Mashed potatoes
- Salad of mixed greens, lightly dressed (1 cup [55 g] greens; 1½ teaspoons [7 g] dressing)
- Mineral water or wine

CHAPTER 7

RECIPES FOR THE LOW-GLYCAL DIET—
A PLAN YOU CAN LIVE WITH

MOSTLY LOW-, SOME MEDIUM-, AND A FEW HIGH-GLYCAL RECIPES

EFFORTLESS WEIGHT LOSS, DELICIOUS MEALS, AND A PLAN YOU CAN LIVE WITH FOR LIFE

This chapter gives you 75 recipes (including variations) that work for following the Low-Glycal Diet, whether you are in Step 1, Step 2 or Step 3 of the plan. These recipes call for easy-to-find ingredients, can be prepared in a typical home kitchen and are delicious and healthful as well as satisfying. We hope you'll try them all and that some will become new favorites.

These recipes fit into the sample meal plans you found in Chapters 4, 5 and 6. They are categorized by meal: breakfast, lunch, dinner, side dishes and snacks, and each recipe lists the calories, GL (glycemic load) and glycals in a single serving. Within each of the meal plans, the page number for every recipe is included so you can turn to it quickly, but you can also look up recipes by name or primary ingredient in the Index at the back of this book.

Most of the recipes here are green (low-glycal) because that is the kind of meal you will be eating most often, no matter which step of the 3-step Low-Glycal Diet plan you are on. Even after you have achieved your desired weight loss and are on the life-long maintenance phase, your week's meal plan will include more green (low-glycal) meals than medium- or high-glycal meals. The other reason most of the recipes in this book are green is that *you won't find any other collection of recipes where the glycal is even a consideration*, and I want you to succeed in achieving and maintaining your ideal weight.

All the recipes are color coded (green, yellow or red) and nearly all include suggestions for what to serve with them. You will also find information on which ingredients can be swapped out or varied to suit your taste; what happens to the GL (glycemic load) and glycal calculation if you add a glass of wine and whether the meal's color will change if it is served as a lunch dish or at dinner. You'll find tips on how to prepare all or some of a recipe in advance, and how to store partially prepared meals. I want to make eating the low-glycal way as easy and enticing as possible!

But, hey, it's your book so make notes on the pages about how to modify the dishes to suit your meal plan. As you become more familiar with the Low-Glycal Diet app (more about that in the next chapter), we hope you'll come up with some of your own recipes or more healthful variations on family favorites. So go ahead, dive in, and spend some time reading the recipes before you make your personal menu plan for the week. Happy cooking—and eating!

COLOR KEY
GREEN
YELLOW
RED

LOW-GLYCAL DIET BREAKFAST RECIPES

The recipes here are easy to shop for and simple to put together. In addition to recipes, this chapter gives you a wealth of tips on the steps you can do ahead so you can store partially prepared meals in your fridge and freezer—making breakfast, lunch and dinner a snap.

As you have seen in all the meal plans, you don't actually *need* a recipe for each breakfast—a meal of a scrambled egg and two slices of bacon, for example, is one you can make without directions! So is a breakfast of a single serving of hot steel-cut oatmeal; simply follow the directions on the box, bag or can the oats came in. Breakfast dishes in the meal plan that *do* require a recipe can be found after the do-ahead short cuts that follow. Simply keep in mind that a breakfast high in protein will provide you with long-lasting energy for the morning and will help you feel full longer.

READY, SET, GO!

No matter what your schedule may be, if you have a week's worth of low-glycal breakfasts (and snacks and lunches!) in your fridge, ready to go to the office, you are off to a great start with the diet. Relax, and enjoy the results!

MISSING THAT TOAST WITH YOUR BACON AND EGGS?

For many of us, toast has been a staple at breakfast our whole lives. But, as you've seen in the meal plans, your low-glycal breakfast of bacon and eggs does not include toast. Fear not: You can *still* have toast (or a bagel) in the low-glycal plan—just make it a mid-morning snack with your coffee or tea. You can even top it with a little peanut or almond butter. Now, your breakfast is low-glycal and so is your snack, and you still get to enjoy toast!

Basic Cheese Omelet with Variations

Can also be served for lunch

A puffy, golden omelet for breakfast is a great low-glycal way to start the day. Eggs and cheese have zero glycals, and the protein provided keeps you full until it's time for a mid-morning snack.

YIELD: 1 SERVING

1 tbsp (15 g) butter

1 egg, well beaten

2 tbsp (28 g) grated cheese (Swiss, cheddar, Fontana, or other firm cheese—your choice)

Salt and freshly ground black pepper

Heat the butter in a 6-inch (15-cm) skillet over medium heat and when the butter is sizzling hot, pour in the beaten egg and tip the pan, if necessary, so that the egg covers the bottom in an even layer. As soon as the egg begins to set, add the grated cheese, sprinkling it evenly over the egg. Let the egg continue to cook a bit before folding the omelet.

Work a spatula under half of the egg, loosening it if it is sticking to the pan, and carefully fold the omelet in half. Lower the heat to medium-low and continue cooking the omelet until it is puffy and golden (about 2 minutes more). Remove from the skillet and season to taste with salt and pepper.

Per Serving: Calories 163 • GL 0 • Glycals 0

VARIATIONS: In place of the cheese, or on top of it, add a small portion (approximately ⅛ cup [10 g]) of any one of the following:

• Spinach, cooked, excess water squeezed out
• Mushrooms, sautéed
• Cherry tomatoes, chopped
• Asparagus tips, steamed

Cheesy Baked Egg

As the information at the end of this recipes shows, this hearty little dish has zero glycals, even when you add bacon. You can assemble a few of these at a time and store them covered and unbaked (or partially cooked) in the fridge until ready to finish.

YIELD: 1 SERVING

½ tbsp (7 g) butter

1 tbsp (7 g) sour cream

1 tsp snipped fresh chives

1 egg

2 tbsp (28 g) grated cheese (Swiss, cheddar or other hard cheese of your choice)

Salt and freshly ground black pepper

Preheat the oven to 350°F (180°C). Melt the butter and pour it into a single-serving oven-proof custard dish. Add the sour cream and spread it out evenly; distribute the chives evenly over the sour cream. Break the egg into the dish, centering the yolk. Place the custard dish in the center of a pie plate. Sprinkle the cheese on the egg, making a wreath around the yolk. Carefully pour warm water into the pie plate until it reaches half an inch (1.3 cm) up the side of the custard dish. Place in the oven and bake for 15 to 20 minutes or until the yolk is set to your preference. Remove from oven; place the custard dish on a rack and let sit for a minute before serving. Eat directly from the custard cup, or run a knife around the edge and transfer to a plate. Season to taste with salt and pepper.

Per Serving: Calories 202 • GL 0 • Glycals 0
With 2 pieces of bacon: Calories 727 • GL 0 • Glycals 0
With bacon and ½ grapefruit: Calories 763 • GL 2 • Glycals 15

Eggs Florentine

Can also be served for brunch

Eggs are a low-glycal star, and so is cheese. More good news: this breakfast recipe can do double-duty as a low-glycal side dish at dinner, too. Easy yet impressive enough for a brunch spread, this yummy combination of eggs, spinach and cheese can be baked in a soufflé dish for an accompaniment to any main course at dinner.

YIELD: 6 SERVINGS

1 (10 oz [280 g]) package frozen chopped spinach

3 eggs, beaten with ¼ cup (60 g) cream

¼ cup (55 g) butter, melted

½ lb (225 g) Swiss cheese, grated

½ lb (225 g) feta cheese, crumbled

Pinch of nutmeg

Salt and freshly ground black pepper

6 eggs, poached

Preheat the oven to 350°F (180°C). Cook the spinach according to the directions on the package. Drain well in a colander, then squeeze between paper towels to remove all moisture. Set aside. Crack the eggs into a large bowl and beat well. Add the melted butter, cheeses, nutmeg, salt and pepper and mix together. Add the spinach and blend until all ingredients are thoroughly combined.

Pour the mixture into 6 greased custard dishes. Bake for 15 to 25 minutes or until puffy and golden on the top. Remove from the oven and let sit on a rack while you poach the eggs.

To serve, release the spinach custard from its dish and center it on a plate, topped with a poached egg.

Per Serving: Calories 271 • GL 0 • Glycals 0

Variation: Spinach Soufflé

For a Spinach Soufflé side dish at dinner, increase the eggs to 4, and bake in a buttered 1 quart (946-ml) soufflé dish for 25 minutes or until puffy and golden.

Eggs Benedict

Can also be served for brunch

This Hollandaise sauce is made in the blender! No double-boiler, no whisking like a fiend to keep the eggs from scrambling—and, it's low-glycal! (English muffins are the only thing that makes this recipe high-glycal.) Try the Hollandaise over asparagus, too.

Have all the ingredients ready to go when you make the Hollandaise sauce because it will be ready very quickly.

YIELD: 4 SERVINGS

4 poached eggs

4 slices Canadian bacon, grilled

4 English muffins, buttered and grilled

HOLLANDAISE SAUCE

3 egg yolks

2 tbsp (28 ml) fresh lemon juice

¼ tsp white pepper

½ cup (112 g) butter, melted

1 tbsp (15 g) fresh chopped chives

To poach eggs, fill a lightly oiled skillet with fresh cold water. Heat the water until it is just about to boil, then lower the heat, and gently crack in the 4 eggs. Once the eggs are in the hot water, adjust the heat so the water is just simmering. Allow the eggs to cook for 3 to 5 minutes.

While the eggs are cooking, butter and grill the English muffins, and cook the Canadian bacon.

Top an English muffin half with a piece of bacon, and then with a poached egg (lift them out of the water with a slotted spoon). Top with a generous pour of Hollandaise, and sprinkle chopped chives over the top. Place the other half of the English muffin on the plate. Serve immediately.

To make the Hollandaise sauce: combine the egg yolks, lemon juice and pepper in a blender, and process for 1 minute. With the blender running, pour in the melted butter, sizzling hot, in a slow, steady stream. Continue blending until the sauce is the desired thickness, usually a couple of minutes.

Per Serving: Calories 906 • GL 11 • Glycals 94

Without the English muffin, this breakfast/brunch dish becomes GREEN

YIELD: 4 SERVINGS
Per Serving: Calories 754 • GL 0 • Glycals 0

Smoked Salmon and Dill Baked Egg

Here's another example of the healthful nature of low-glycal eating. Salmon, which has a zero GL and glycal profile, is an excellent source of omega-3, a fatty acid that promotes cardiac health as well as eye, skin and brain health. Smoked salmon will keep well in your freezer, allowing you to have it on hand to use as needed. It adds a delicious briny, butter complement to eggs, and dill and salmon are a classic pairing that never loses its appeal.

YIELD: 1 SERVING

½ tbsp (7 g) butter

1 tbsp (15 g) sour cream

½ tsp chopped fresh dill

1 egg

2 slices smoked salmon (approximately 4 oz [115 g])

Salt and freshly ground black pepper to taste

Preheat the oven to 350°F (180°C). Butter a single-serving oven-proof custard dish. Add the sour cream and spread it to make an even layer. Add the chopped fresh dill. Break the egg into the dish, centering the yolk. Place the custard dish in the center of a pie plate. Carefully pour warm water into the pie plate until it reaches half an inch (1.3 cm) up the side of the custard dish. Place in the oven and bake for 15 to 20 minutes or until the yolk is set to your preference. Remove from the oven; place the custard dish on a rack and let sit for 1 minute. Place the smoked salmon on a breakfast plate. Run a knife around the edge of the baked egg and holding the custard dish with a pot holder (it will be hot) tip the egg out onto the salmon. Season to taste with salt and freshly ground black pepper.

Per Serving: Calories 224 • GL 0 • Glycals 0

Asparagus Frittata

Can also be served for lunch or dinner

Frittata is a variation on an omelet and omelets are a terrific low-glycal breakfast, lunch or even dinner. If you prepare it for dinner and have leftovers, you can enjoy it again the next day as a satisfying lunch. No need to reheat it, either—simply allow it to come to room temperature and serve it with a green salad.

As with omelets, the variations on this frittata are nearly endless. When asparagus is not available, you can substitute steamed broccoli, sautéed Swiss chard or spinach, sliced sautéed zucchini, strips of roasted red bell pepper—or whatever is in season—with no significant change in the glycemic load or glycals.

YIELD: 4 SERVINGS

---

1 lb (455 g) asparagus (about 15 stalks)

2 tsp (10 ml) olive oil

1 small onion, thinly sliced

½ teaspoon salt

4 eggs, lightly beaten

1 cup (120 g) shredded Swiss or Gruyère cheese

1 pinch freshly ground black pepper

Variation: Zucchini Frittata

Substitute 2 small zucchini (split lengthwise and cut into ¼ inch [6-mm] slices) for the asparagus; sauté until tender and slightly browned. And substitute ¾ cup (75 g) grated Parmesan cheese for the Swiss or Gruyère cheese.

Preheat broiler. Snap off and discard the tough ends of each asparagus spear. Cut the spears diagonally into 1 inch (2.5-cm) lengths. Set aside. Place the oil in a 10 inch (25.4-cm) ovenproof skillet set over medium-high heat. When the oil is hot but not smoking add the onion and sprinkle with salt. Lower the heat to medium-low and cook, stirring occasionally, until the onions are softened but not browned, about 2 to 3 minutes.

Add the asparagus to the skillet and reduce the heat to low. Cover and cook for about 5 to 6 minutes, or until the asparagus is barely tender.

Pour the beaten eggs into the skillet and leave over the heat for another 2 minutes or until the eggs are almost set but still runny on top.

Sprinkle the cheese evenly over the eggs. Remove the skillet from the top of the stove and transfer to a rack set about 4 inches (10.2 cm) below the broiler. Watch closely! Broil only until the cheese is melted and brown, about 2 minutes depending on your boiler.

Run a spatula around the edge of the frittata to loosen it from the pan and carefully slide it onto a large serving platter. Let it sit for 2 minutes, then cut into wedges. Serve hot or at room temperature.

Per Serving: Calories 224 • GL 0 • Glycals 1

Sausage Frittata

This frittata is only low-glycal for breakfast or lunch; at dinner, it becomes medium-glycal, which is OK if you've planned for a yellow (medium-glycal) dinner. Add a small green salad and you've got a healthful and tasty meal that's quick and economical.

This recipe makes a breakfast of sausage and eggs easy to take to work; cut into wedges and you are good to go.

YIELD: 4 SERVINGS

1 tbsp (15 g) butter

2 shallots, thinly sliced (or half an onion, thinly sliced)

¾ lb (340 g) sausage meat (pork or turkey)

4 eggs, well beaten

1 tbsp (15 ml) milk

Salt and freshly ground black pepper to taste

3 tbsp (15 g) grated Parmesan cheese

Preheat oven to 350°F (180°C). Melt the butter in an oven-proof 8-inch (20.3-cm) skillet set over medium heat. Add the shallot and cook for 1 minute. Add the sausage, crumbled; cook, stirring, until browned. Meanwhile, combine the beaten eggs with the milk and season to taste with salt and freshly ground black pepper. Pour the egg mixture into the skillet, over the sausage. Sprinkle the grated cheese over the top. Remove from the heat and place in the preheated oven. Bake for approximately 12 to 15 minutes or until the eggs are set and the top of the frittata is puffy and golden. Remove from the oven and let sit for 2 minutes. Slice into 4 wedges and serve hot or at room temperature.

Per Serving (pork sausage): Calories 421 • GL 2 • Glycals 10

Broiled Tomatoes

Can also be served for breakfast, brunch or a dinner side dish

A juicy broiled tomato makes a great low-glycal complement to just about any egg dish at breakfast, and also goes well with a steak, chop or baked fish. The better the tomato, the better the results, but the garlic, cheese and parsley in this recipe can "improve" a less-than-perfect tomato.

YIELD: 8 SERVINGS

---

4 large ripe tomatoes

2 tbsp (30 ml) olive oil

Salt and pepper, to taste

1 garlic clove, minced

½ cup (25 g) grated Parmesan cheese

4 tbsp (55 g) butter, cubed

¼ cup (15 g) fresh chopped flat leaf parsley

Preheat broiler. Wash the tomatoes, and halve each, cutting through the stem end. Set on paper towels, cut side down, for about 20 minutes.

Place the tomatoes, cut side up, in a shallow casserole dish. Brush the tops with olive oil. Season with salt, pepper and garlic. Sprinkle with cheese, and dot with butter. Sprinkle with chopped parsley.

Place the baking dish under the broiler until the cheese is bubbly and browned, approximately 3 minutes. *Watch closely so as not to burn*! Serve immediately.

Per Serving: Calories 132 • GL 1 • Glycals 1

LOW-GLYCAL DIET LUNCH RECIPES

The recipes here are easy to shop for and, for the most part, simple to put together. While you are welcome to stick with your favorite low-glycal lunch Monday thru Friday (or every day, for that matter) if that suits you, it's nice to have other options.

Many of these lunches are suitable for dinner, too, so be sure to check them out with that in mind. And, because nearly every recipe in this section is green (low-glycal), you'll be greatly expanding your low-glycal dinner options.

Remember, you can use the app to create more lunch favorites.

Asian Chicken Salad

Chicken is a versatile low-glycal ingredient. As a salad, it makes such a satisfying brown-bag lunch for the office, it's good to have a few variations on the theme. Here, fresh ginger, garlic and hot pepper flakes give it a new twist; the lettuce and bean sprouts add crunch. You can substitute seared scallops for the chicken for excellent results.

YIELD: 4 SERVINGS

DRESSING

¼ cup (60 ml) rice wine vinegar

1 tbsp (15 ml) soy sauce

2 tbsp (30 ml) vegetable oil

¼ tsp sesame oil

1 tbsp (8 g) grated fresh ginger

1 garlic clove, minced

¼ tsp red pepper flakes

2 cups (110 g) chopped iceberg lettuce

1 cup (50 g) mung bean sprouts

2 chicken breast, boneless, skinless, cooked and shredded

1 carrot, shredded

2 scallions, thinly sliced

Make the dressing by combining the vinegar, soy sauce, vegetable oil, sesame oil, ginger, garlic and red pepper flakes. Whisk until well mixed.

Place the chopped lettuce, bean sprouts, shredded chicken, carrots and scallions in a large bowl; pour the dressing over all and toss well. Divide between 4 plates and serve.

Per Serving: Calories 210 • GL 2 • Glycals 6

Caprese Salad

Can also be served for dinner

Tomatoes have a low-glycemic load and low-glycal count. Mozzarella cheese has zero GL and zero glycals. Together, in this traditional dish from Capri, they make a tasty low-glycal salad, whether served at lunch or dinner. Add a protein like tuna or swordfish and you have a satisfying meal. Make this salad when tomatoes and basil are at their peak, purchased from a farmers' market or road-side stand—or plucked from your own garden.

YIELD: 4 SERVINGS

---

6 large ripe tomatoes, cut crossways into ¼" (6-mm) slices

1 lb (455 g) fresh mozzarella, cut into ¼" (6-mm) slices

6 tbsp (90 ml) extra-virgin olive oil

3 tbsp (45 ml) balsamic vinegar

Salt and freshly ground black pepper to taste

8–12 fresh basil leaves

Arrange the slices of tomato and cheese on a large platter, alternating them in a decorative pattern.

In a bowl, whisk together the olive oil, vinegar, salt and pepper. Drizzle the dressing over the tomato and mozzarella slices.

Cut the fresh basil leaves into thin strips and sprinkle them over the dish. Serve immediately.

Per Serving: Calories 417 • GL 2 • Glycals 6
Add canned or grilled tuna (¼ lb [115 g] per person):
Calories 700 • GL 1 • Glycals 10

FOR DINNER:
Add grilled swordfish (½ lb [225 g] per person):
Calories 625 • GL 1 • Glycals 9
❢ Add a glass of white wine: Calories 724 • GL 1 • Glycals 10

Cobb Salad

Can also be served for dinner

In a Cobb salad, all the starring ingredients are low-glycal, and they remain that way when combined. The chicken, avocado, tomato, egg, bacon and cheese are sliced, chopped or crumbled to be about the same size and then arranged in bands across a bed of chopped, crisp greens, making a striking presentation. When you dig in, the uniform small pieces of the ingredients makes for a very pleasant mouthful of flavors all at once. It takes a bit of time to prep and assemble this salad but the good news is you can cover it carefully with plastic wrap and store in the fridge for a couple of hours before serving—helpful when you're hosting a party.

YIELD: 6 SERVINGS

DRESSING

3 tbsp (45 ml) red wine vinegar

1 tbsp (15 ml) fresh lemon juice

2 tsp (10 g) Dijon mustard

1 garlic clove, minced

½ tsp salt

½ tsp black pepper

½ cup (120 ml) extra-virgin olive oil

½ head romaine lettuce, chopped (3 cups [165 g])

½ head iceberg lettuce, chopped (3 cups [165 g])

2 ripe avocados, halved, peeled, and cut into ½" (1.3-cm) cubes

6 bacon slices, cooked until crisp, drained on paper towels and crumbled

3 chicken breasts (skinless boneless), cooked and cut into bite-size cubes

3 medium tomatoes, cut into ½" (1.3-cm) cubes

¾ cup (90 g) Roquefort cheese (or your favorite blue cheese), crumbled

3 eggs, hard-boiled and chopped

¼ cup (4 g) finely chopped chives

Make the dressing: In a bowl, whisk together the vinegar, lemon juice, mustard, garlic, salt and pepper. Add the oil slowly, whisking until emulsified. Set aside. Toss together the Romaine and iceberg lettuce; place in an even layer on a platter. Top with the remaining ingredients, arranged in bands. Set on the table and let your guests admire it. Just before serving, pour half of the dressing over the salad and toss gently. Pour the remainder of the dressing over the salad and serve.

Note: You can also assemble this salad in layers in a straight-sided clear glass salad bowl (a trifle bowl works well for this), starting with the lettuce followed by the chicken, bacon, tomato, cheese, avocado, egg and chives. This makes for a pretty presentation and you may find it easier. Bring the bowl to the table to let your guests admire it; just before serving, pour the dressing over the salad and toss gently.

If you are not making this for a party and don't care about arranging the ingredients in bands or layers, simply place all the ingredients in a large bowl, add the dressing, toss together and serve.

Per Serving: Calories 675 • GL 1 • Glycals 6
❢ Add a glass of white wine: Calories 774 • GL 1 • Glycals 7

FOR DINNER:
❢ Add a glass of wine: no change from lunch to the calories, GL or glycals
At dinner you can increase the chicken to a full serving (1 breast), ❢ include a glass of wine, and still have a green meal:
Calories 885 • GL 1 • Glycals 8

Clam Chowder

Clams, like all seafood, are low GL and low-glycal. Making clam chowder yourself means you can leave out the potatoes—not the case in restaurants or in canned chowder. The addition of potatoes would change this chowder from low-glycal to high-glycal. You won't miss them, though; chock-full of clams in a flavorful broth, this chowder is bound to become your favorite.

YIELD: 4 SERVINGS

2 pieces thick-sliced bacon, cut into small pieces

½ cup (80 g) chopped onion

¼ cup (25 g) minced celery

Salt and freshly ground black pepper

2 cups (475 ml) clam juice

2 (6.5-oz [184-g]) cans chopped clams

1½ cups (355 ml) milk

1 tsp dried thyme

1 tbsp (14 g) butter

2 tbsp (8 g) minced fresh flat leaf parsley

In a heavy-bottomed soup pot set over medium heat, cook the bacon until crisp. Remove the bacon with a slotted spoon, and set it aside. Pour off all but 1 tablespoon (15 g) of the rendered fat, add the onion and celery and cook over medium-low heat until the onion is tender and translucent but not browned. Season with salt and pepper. Add the clam juice; stir and bring to a simmer. Cover the pot partially with a lid and simmer for 5 minutes.

Add the clams, milk, thyme and reserved cooked bacon. Stir, cover the pot and set the heat to the lowest setting. Check it in a couple of minutes and turn off the heat when the mixture begins to simmer. Add the butter and parsley; stir, and serve.

Per Serving: Calories 210 • GL 1 • Glycals 2

Crabmeat and Avocado Salad

Can also be served for dinner

Crabmeat is a versatile low-glycal shellfish that can be enjoyed in hot or cold dishes, which is why you'll find a number of recipes in this book that call for it. If you can purchase fresh crabmeat, do. But, fresh-frozen crabmeat or canned crabmeat can be just as good and either way you get omega-3 fatty acids and calcium. With canned, you get what you pay for; so don't go for the least expensive brand. Of course, if you've had a crab boil and have leftovers, use that meat for the salad.

The creamy texture and delicate flavor of avocado let the sweet flavor of the crab take center stage.

YIELD: 4 SERVINGS

---

2 cups (270 g) lump white crabmeat, fresh or canned (drained, if canned)

2 tbsp (28 g) minced celery

2 tbsp (6 g) chopped fresh chives

⅓ cup (75 g) mayonnaise

1 tbsp (15 ml) fresh lemon juice

Salt and pepper to taste

4 large Bibb lettuce leaves

2 scallions, thinly sliced (white and light green part only)

2 ripe avocados, halved, peeled, pitted and sliced

Place the crab, celery and chives in a bowl, and toss lightly to combine. In a separate bowl, whisk together the mayonnaise, lemon juice, and salt and pepper. Pour the dressing over the crab mixture and combine well.

Place a lettuce leaf on each of 4 salad plates. Scoop about ½ cup (70 g) of the crabmeat salad onto each lettuce leaf. Sprinkle each serving with a portion of the green onions. Arrange the sliced avocado on the side of the crabmeat salad. Serve immediately.

Per Serving: Calories 451 • GL 1 • Glycals 3

FOR DINNER:
Per Serving: Calories 451 • GL 1 • Glycals 3
❢ Add a glass of white wine: Calories 550 • GL 1 • Glycals 4

Curried Shrimp Salad

Can also be served for dinner

Good news, shrimp lovers: this readily available shellfish is low-glycal, and can be prepared in a multitude of ways that keep it low-glycal. Curry makes a good match for it and adds a pleasant heat to this chilled salad. This dish tastes even better if it's allowed to sit for a while; so make it a day ahead if you can.

YIELD: 2 SERVINGS

6-8 jumbo shrimp, boiled in their shells, cooled, peeled and deveined

¼ cup (25 g) minced celery

2 scallions, very finely sliced

½ cup (115 g) plain yogurt

2 tbsp (28 g) mayonnaise

1 tsp curry powder

Salt and freshly ground black pepper, to taste

2 tbsp (2 g) chopped fresh cilantro

Place the shrimp in a large bowl. In a separate bowl, combine the celery, scallions, yogurt, mayonnaise and curry powder. Stir together well and season the mixture to taste with salt and pepper; pour the dressing over the shrimp and toss gently to coat them evenly. Cover and store in fridge until ready to serve. Best if left overnight or for at least 2 hours.

Remove the curried shrimp from the fridge, toss and place a single portion on a bed of salad greens (approximately 1 cup [55 g] of torn Romaine or other crisp lettuce per person). Sprinkle with fresh cilantro and serve.

Per Serving: Calories 385 • GL 3 • Glycals 12

Egg Salad

Eggs are a low-glycal diet staple for any meal of the day. They are a zero glycal and zero glycemic load food, and they are an excellent source of vitamin B-12 and other important nutrients. Versatile and economical, you'll want to have them on hand at all times. Egg salad can be taken to work as lunch; enjoy it over a bed of chopped crisp iceberg lettuce, or with tender tangy watercress. Or, try one of the variations below, wrap in Boston lettuce and enjoy an egg salad roll-up.

YIELD: 2 SERVINGS.

4 hard-boiled eggs, cooled and shelled

3 tbsp (42 g) mayonnaise

½ tsp Dijon mustard

Salt and freshly ground black pepper to taste

Run the hard-boiled eggs through an egg slicer twice, or chop them by hand. Place in a bowl and add the mayonnaise, mustard and salt and pepper to taste. Mix well. Cover and chill.

Per Serving: Calories 334 • GL 0 • Glycals 0

VARIATIONS:

Herbed Egg Salad: add to the mix ½ teaspoon dried tarragon, or 1 teaspoon chopped fresh tarragon. Or add 2 teaspoons (2 g) of finely snipped fresh chives or flat leaf parsley.

Egg Salad with Cherry Tomatoes: add to the mix ¼ cup (38 g) finely chopped cherry tomatoes and 1 teaspoon minced fresh marjoram.

Egg Salad & Ham: add to the mix ¼ cup (38 g) finely chopped baked ham.

Egg Salad Roll-Ups: Place 2 generous tablespoons (30 g) of egg salad on a leaf of Boston lettuce and roll into a wrap.

Eggplant Salad

Can also be served for a dinner side dish

You can eat meat without a thought on the Low-Glycal Diet because meat is low-glycal. But you'll want to eat vegetables, too—because you like them and because your body needs them. Eggplant and the other vegetables here fit the low-glycal bill and, as you can see in the serving suggestions at the end of the recipe, this side dish makes a tasty low-glycal meal with fish or meat.

Make this salad in the morning to enjoy later that afternoon or evening. For lunch, serve on a bed of torn crisp Romaine lettuce. However you serve it, you'll love the combination of tender eggplant, juicy tomato, crisp red pepper, and savory Kalamata olives pulled together with an herbed dressing and crumbled feta cheese.

YIELD: 4 SERVINGS

---

1 large eggplant, cut into ½" (1.3-cm) cubes

DRESSING

5 tbsp (75 ml) olive oil

2 tbsp (30 ml) red wine vinegar

1 garlic clove, minced

¼ tsp dried thyme

¼ tsp dried oregano

1 tbsp (15 ml) lemon juice

Salt and black pepper

¼ cup (15 g) chopped flat leaf parsley

1 red bell pepper, minced

1 cup (150 g) cherry tomatoes, chopped

½ cup (50 g) pitted Greek olives, rough chopped

1 cup (150 g) crumbled feta cheese

Preheat oven to 375°F (190°C). Coat a shallow baking pan with 1 tablespoon (15 ml) of the olive oil. Spread the eggplant cubes onto the pan, and toss so that each piece is lightly coated with oil. Bake for approximately 10 to 15 minutes, or until the cubes are tender (test one with a fork). Remove from oven and transfer pan to a cooling rack.

While the eggplant is cooling, in a large bowl whisk together the remaining olive oil, vinegar, garlic, dried herbs, lemon juice and salt and pepper to taste. Add the warm eggplant cubes and toss well. Cover the bowl with plastic wrap and let sit at room temperature for 2 hours.

An hour before you are ready to serve the salad, add the parsley, red pepper, cherry tomatoes and olives to the eggplant. Toss together gently. Top each serving with crumbled feta cheese.

Per Serving (without lettuce): Calories 150 • GL 2 • Glycals 2
Per Serving (with lettuce): Calories 156 • GL 2 • Glycals 3
Add a pan-fried flounder fillet: Calories 267 • GL 2 • Glycals 4

FOR DINNER:
With a lamb chop and small green salad: Calories 571 • GL 2 • Glycals 9
❢ Add a glass of red wine: Calories 673 • GL 2 • Glycals 11

Lobster Salad

Can also be served for dinner

Lobster might be a pocketbook spurge but it's not a diet splurge, at least not on the Low-Glycal Diet—on its own it's a zero glycal and zero GL food. (Even dipped in melted butter, lobster keeps its zero status.) A lobster salad is a great way to use up extra lobster meat the day after a steamed lobster dinner. Or, you can buy cooked lobster meat at your fish market; it will cost more per pound but does save you the work of cooking the lobsters and picking the meat. In this rendition, celery adds crunch, and the flat leaf parsley brings out the flavor of the lemon juice in the dressing.

YIELD: 4 SERVINGS

1 lb (455 g) cooked lobster meat, coarsely chopped

½ cup (25 g) finely diced celery

2 tbsp (8 g) finely chopped fresh flat leaf parsley

½ cup (115 g) mayonnaise

1 tbsp (15 ml) fresh lemon juice

Salt and freshly ground black pepper

1 head Boston lettuce or other tender-leaf lettuce

2 large tomatoes, cut into wedges

1 European cucumber, sliced

In a large bowl, combine the lobster meat with the celery and parsley. Toss. Add the mayonnaise, lemon juice, salt and pepper. Toss to combine. Cover and refrigerate.

To serve, place a few leaves of Boston lettuce on each plate. Spoon a mound of lobster salad into the middle of the lettuce. Surround the lobster salad with tomato wedges and cucumber slices.

Per Serving: Calories 423 • GL 4 • Glycals 18

Salade Niçoise

Can also be served for dinner

The only traditional ingredient missing from this classic salad/meal-in-one dish: boiled potatoes. The addition of potatoes takes this low-glycal meal to high-glycal, but you won't even miss them. Named for the small purple-black olive that is only one of its many ingredients, this hearty salad is an excellent choice for a leisurely summer weekend lunch or dinner. A number of variations on this classic French dish exist; true to its Mediterranean origins, this one calls for the always-key ingredients of tuna, anchovy, green beans, hard-boiled egg and—of course—olives. At lunch, add a glass of dry white wine and you will still have a green meal—and at dinner, too.

YIELD: 4 SERVINGS

DRESSING

3 tbsp (45 ml) cider vinegar

2 tbsp (30 ml) finely minced shallots

1 tbsp (15 ml) Dijon mustard

8 tbsp (120 ml) olive oil

1 anchovy, mashed

1 tbsp (4 g) finely chopped fresh flat leaf parsley

1 tbsp (4 g) finely chopped fresh tarragon

Salt and pepper

4 cups (220 g) Bibb lettuce leaves, roughly torn, tightly packed

16 oz (455 g) tuna packed in olive oil (Italian-style is best for this dish)

½ lb (225 g) green beans, blanched,* cooled and stem ends trimmed

2 hard-boiled eggs, shelled and quartered

½ cup (50 g) Niçoise olives, pitted (Kalamata olives are a good substitute)

In a small bowl, stir together the vinegar and shallots; whisk in the mustard. Add the olive oil in a slow stream, whisking constantly, until the mixture is emulsified. Mix in the anchovy and season to taste with salt and pepper. Whisk in the fresh herbs and set aside.

To assemble the salad: divide the lettuce between 4 plates. Top each serving with a portion of tuna, green beans, hard-boiled egg and olives. Drizzle a little dressing over each, or serve the dressing on the side in a small pitcher.

*To blanch the green beans: Bring 2 quarts (1.9 L) of lightly salted water to a boil. Add the green beans, cover and as soon as the water returns to a boil remove the cover and cook for 2 minutes. Drain into a colander and allow to cool.

Per Serving: Calories 679 • GL 1 • Glycals 5

🍷 Add a glass of white wine: Calories 778 • GL 1 • Glycals 6

Salmon Salad Wraps

If you are accustomed to taking a sandwich to work every day for lunch, you need some fresh ideas to go low-glycal. Virtually anything you can put between two slices of bread can be wrapped in a tender lettuce leaf instead. Like all seafood, salmon is a zero glycal/ zero GL food, and it's a great source of healthful protein and omega-3 fatty acids. You can make this dish with leftover broiled, baked or poached salmon fillets, or you can use canned salmon. The cucumber adds a pleasing crunch to the mixture.

YIELD: 2 SERVINGS

2 cups (260 g) flaked cooked salmon (if using canned salmon, drain off the liquid)

¾ cup (90 g) seeded, finely diced cucumber (unpeeled; English cucumbers are a good choice)

1 tbsp (3 g) chopped fresh chives

2 tbsp (28 g) mayonnaise

1 tsp fresh lemon juice

Salt and pepper to taste

6 large Boston lettuce (or other "butter" lettuce) leaves

Place the salmon, cucumber and chives in a medium-size bowl and toss together lightly. In a separate bowl, whisk together the mayonnaise, lemon juice, and salt and pepper. Pour the dressing over the salmon mixture and toss gently.

Arrange the lettuce leaves on a flat surface and place equal portions of the salmon salad on each one. Wrap and fold the lettuce securely around the filling and place (with the outside edge of the leaf facing down) on two plates and serve.

Per Serving: Calories 452 • GL 2 • Glycals 11

Sirloin and Black Bean Burrito

Can also be served for dinner

Here, a leaf of Romaine lettuce takes the place of the traditional flour tortilla, transforming a high-glycal meal to low-glycal. But you still get a delicious combo of steak, beans, and guacamole in every bite! During Step 2 or Step 3 of the diet, you can swap out the lettuce for flour tortillas because you can have one red (high-glycal) meal a week while you follow Step 2; in Step 3, one day a week allows *all* red meals.

YIELD: 4 SERVINGS (2 BURRITOS PER PERSON)

1 cup (170 g) cooked black beans (if canned, rinsed), mashed and warm

1 large garlic clove, smashed with ¼ tsp salt

8 Romaine lettuce leaves, large

1 (1 lb [455 g]) grilled sirloin steak, thinly sliced

1 cup (115 g) shredded cheese (cheddar or Monterey jack)

1 cup (225 g) guacamole (recipe on page 170)

1 cup (260 g) tomato salsa, or as needed

In a small skillet over low heat, mix the garlic and salt into the black beans.

Select 8 of the best large outer leaves from a head of Romaine lettuce. Clean and set on a work surface.

Place a few slices of steak on each leaf of Romaine. Top the steak with a portion of beans, cheese, guacamole and salsa. Roll as if making a burrito with a flour tortilla. Serve 2 per person with extra salsa on the side.

Per Serving: Calories 287 • GL 3 • Glycals 8

Tarragon Chicken Salad

Can also be served for dinner

Like eggs, chicken is a versatile, economical low-glycal food that can be made into a nearly endless variety of hot or cold dishes. Here's one that's suitable for lunch or dinner, no matter which step of the diet you're on. As with any chicken salad, you can start with a cooked rotisserie chicken to save time. Or, if you prefer, buy fresh chicken and roast or boil it—whole, breasts, tenders, thighs—whichever cut you prefer. Any extra meat can be stored in your fridge or freezer for another meal. When making chicken salad, always remove and discard the skin after cooking.

The combination of fresh and dried tarragon is a bit unusual but you'll find it greatly enhances the flavor of the salad, and the sour cream keeps the mayonnaise from masking the delicate taste of the herb. If you don't have fresh tarragon on hand, increase the dried amount by 1 teaspoon—it will still be delicious!

(By the way, you can use turkey for this recipe, if you prefer).

YIELD: 4 SERVINGS

4 cups (560 g) cubed cooked chicken meat (breast meat)

1½ cups (150 g) diced celery

1 tbsp (4 g) finely chopped fresh tarragon

⅔ cup (77 g) sour cream

½ cup (115 g) mayonnaise

1 tbsp (4.8 g) dried tarragon

½ tsp salt

¼ tsp freshly ground pepper

8 Boston lettuce (or other tender lettuce) leaves

In a large bowl, combine the chicken, celery and fresh tarragon. In a separate bowl, whisk together the sour cream, mayonnaise, dried tarragon and salt and pepper. Pour the dressing over the chicken mixture and toss to coat evenly. Cover the bowl with plastic wrap and refrigerate for at least 1 hour to allow flavor to develop.

Serve each portion on a bed of 2 large lettuce leaves.

Per Serving: Calories 434 • GL 0 • Glycals 2
❢ Add a glass of white wine:
Per Serving: Calories 533 • GL 0 • Glycals 2
Add 1 cup (150 g) of halved seedless red grapes to the recipe
Per Serving: Calories 551 • GL 3 • Glycals 14

FOR DINNER:
Per Serving: Calories 434 • GL 0 • Glycals 2
Add a serving (6 spears) of steamed asparagus and you have
Per Serving: Calories 572 • GL 1 • Glycals 6 or
Add a fresh sliced tomato or cup of cherry tomatoes, halved
Per Serving: Calories 590 • GL 0 • Glycals 11
❢ Add a glass of white wine:
Per Serving: Calories 689 • GL 1 • Glycals 12

Tuna Salad Plate or Roll-ups

Canned tuna is a great staple of the Low-Glycal Diet because on its own (1) it's a zero GL/zero glycal food and, (2) it's easily stored in your cupboard (it's also a great source of omega-3 fatty acids—good for your heart, skin, and brain). But, put tuna salad between two pieces of bread and you suddenly have a high-glycal meal. The solution: serve the tuna salad on a bed of greens or rolled in lettuce leaves. If tuna salad roll-ups are on your meal plan for lunch at the office, carry the tuna salad in a separate container and make the wraps right before you will eat them; otherwise, the roll-up can become a bit soggy by lunch time.

YIELD: 1 SERVING

1 (5-oz [140-g]) can tuna packed in olive oil, drained

2 tbsp (30 g) minced celery

1 small pickle, chopped (to equal approx. 1 tbsp [15 g])

1 tbsp (14 g) mayonnaise

½ tsp mustard (optional)

4 large Boston lettuce leaves to serve as a bed or as wraps

In a bowl, combine the tuna with all the other ingredients except the lettuce, using a fork to mix evenly. Gently flatten the lettuce leaves and spoon an equal portion of tuna salad on each one. Starting at one end, roll up the layers to make a fat cigar-shaped bundle. Secure with a toothpick, if desired.

Per Serving: Calories 344 • GL 0 • Glycals 1

Vegetable Soup

Sure, you can buy vegetable soup but most brands include potatoes or pasta, either of which turn a low-glycal dish into one that's high-glycal. Plus, making a pot of soup is a great way to use up a few odds and ends languishing in the fridge and this recipe is no exception. Once you've prepped the vegetables for this recipe, your work is done; lower the heat to simmer, set a timer and pick up that newspaper.

YIELD: 4 SERVINGS

2 tbsp (30 ml) olive oil

1 small onion, cut in ¼" (6-mm) dice

½ cup (75 g) finely minced red bell pepper (or cut into matchsticks)

½ cup (35 g) chopped mushrooms (white buttons are fine)

2 carrots, peeled, halved lengthwise and cut into ¼" (6-mm) slices

2 celery stalks, cut in ¼" (6-mm) dice

Salt and pepper

1 tsp dried marjoram

1 bay leaf

1 (14.5-oz [411-g]) can diced tomatoes with liquid

1¾ cups (414 ml) chicken stock

1¼ cups (295 ml) tomato-vegetable juice cocktail

1 cup (235 ml) water

1 cup (100 g) chopped fresh green beans (cut into 1" [2.5-cm] pieces)

In a large stockpot, heat the oil over medium heat and when it is hot, but not smoking, add the onion, red pepper, mushrooms, carrots and celery. Stir with a wooden spoon so that all the ingredients are coated with a bit of oil, season with a pinch of salt and pepper and add the marjoram (rubbing it between your palms over the soup pot). Reduce the heat to low and cover the pot. Lift the lid and stir the vegetables every minute or so until they are tender but not browned; this should take 3 to 5 minutes.

Add the bay leaf, stir and add the diced tomatoes. Increase the heat to medium-high.

As soon as the mixture starts to simmer, add the chicken stock, vegetable juice and water. Stir and return the lid to the pot, set to partially cover it.

Keep an eye on the soup and as soon as it begins to boil reduce the heat to low. Cook, covered, at a low simmer for 20 minutes. Add the green beans and continue cooking at a simmer for another 10 minutes.

Per Serving: Calories 132 • GL 4 • Glycals 5

LOW-GLYCAL DIET DINNER RECIPES

The recipes here are easy to shop for and, for the most part, simple to put together. But, even the dishes that are a bit time-consuming to make are worth trying. And, in many of the recipes here you'll find tips that allow you to make part of the dish in advance so that when it's time to make the meal you can pull it together quickly.

Some of these dinner dishes are suitable for a weekend lunch, too—like the Seafood Chowder—which means your mix-and-match low-glycal meal plans continue to expand. Many of them will provide you with leftovers, too, such as the Sirloin Roast, Whole Roasted Chicken or Flank Steak to name a few, which can become part of a tasty low-glycal lunch the next day.

While some of the recipes here are rich (suitable for cold weather or a special occasion) and others are light (suitable for hot weather or when you're in the mood for lighter fare), nearly every recipe in this section is green (low-glycal). You can make them yellow (medium-glycal) or red (high-glycal), if you like, by adding a side dish or ingredient that changes the glycal status (think: potatoes, rice, pasta or bread) when that suits your menu. Of course, you can also change a green or yellow dinner to yellow or red by adding a dessert, like a dish of fruit sorbet. The beauty of following the Low-Glycal Diet is its flexibility. And remember, you can use the app to create new dinner favorites.

COOKING FOR ONE?

If you are a household of one, you will find that you have a serving or more left over after most meals made from the recipes found here. Consider that scenario a bonus: Package any extra portions to have as lunches during the work week, or for the freezer if it's a dish that freezes well. If you are cooking for one, you can also quite easily change a recipe that serves four into one that serves two, and so on.

Basic Baked, Broiled or Pan-Fried Fish Fillets or Steaks

This chapter contains plenty of recipes for seafood, but it's important to know how to cook a plain piece of fish quickly and simply because seafood is a low-glycal food—usually yielding a zero glycal and zero GL meal, depending on what you pair with it. A serving is generally about 6 to 8 ounces (170–225 g) per person. You can jazz up any of these techniques by adding a splash of white wine as the fish cooks, and a sprinkle of capers and fresh herbs just before the fish is done, or topping the cooked fish with herbed butter* or anchovy butter* as you serve it. Serve with lemon wedges.

BAKED FISH (FILLET OR STEAK)

Preheat oven to 350°F (180°C). Lightly oil a baking dish and place the fillets or steak/s in the pan. Season with a little salt and pepper and a dot of butter (approximately 1 teaspoon). Bake fillets for about 20 minutes, or until flakey. Fish steaks (salmon, tuna, swordfish) will take a little longer, usually about 30 minutes. Serve immediately.

BROILED FISH (FILLET OR STEAK)

Preheat broiler. Set oven rack approx. 6 inches (15.2 cm) below broiler. Lightly oil a broiler pan and set it below broiler until it is hot. Place the fillets or steak/s on it. Season with a little salt and pepper and a dot of butter (approximately 1 teaspoon). Place under the broiler so that the fish is approximately 5 inches (12.7 cm) below the heat. For thin fillets, like flounder, about 7 minutes without turning it should cook the fish nicely. To broil a fish steak, you will flip it after about 4 minutes and continue cooking it for another 5 minutes or until the meat is flakey and cooked. Serve immediately.

PAN-FRIED FISH (FILLET OR STEAK)

Use a cast iron skillet if possible. Add a tablespoon (15 ml) of olive oil and a tablespoon (14 g) of butter to the skillet and heat over medium heat until the butter is sizzling but not browned. Lay the fillets or steak in the skillet. Cook fillets about 3 minutes per side, flipping carefully only once. Cook the steak/s about 4 minutes per side, flipping carefully only once. The fish is done when the meat is flakey and juicy. Serve immediately.

Basic Baked, Broiled or
Pan-Fried Fish Fillets or Steaks (continued)

*HERBED BUTTER
Mix 4 tablespoons (56 g) of softened butter with 1 finely minced garlic clove, 2 tablespoons
(8 g) of mixed finely chopped fresh herbs of your choice such as flat leaf parsley, chives,
tarragon, basil, marjoram or cilantro; add salt and freshly ground black pepper to taste. Chill.
Place a teaspoon of the butter on top of each fillet or steak right before serving.

*ANCHOVY BUTTER
Mix 4 tablespoons (56 g) of softened butter with 1 finely minced shallot, 1 smashed anchovy
fillet, and 1 tablespoon (4 g) of finely chopped fresh flat leaf parsley. Chill. Place a teaspoon
of the butter on top of each fillet or steak right before serving.

Per Serving: Calories will vary (a cod fillet is 137) • GL 0 • Glycals 0
With a green salad: Calories 169 • GL 0 • Glycals 0
❢ Add a glass of white wine: Calories 268 • GL 0 • Glycals 0

Basic Pan-Grilled or Broiled Steaks and Chops

Knowing how to cook a steak or chop simply and quickly is a basic cooking skill that will serve you well on the Low-Glycal Diet. Steaks or chops of beef, pork or lamb are satisfying, healthful low-GL/glycal foods that can be cooked on top of the stove in a grill pan, or under the broiler. Both methods are quick, but if you are using a broiler, keep an eye on it as they can be surprisingly fast.

A single serving is approximately 6 to 8 ounces (170–225 g). The times below are based on boneless steaks or chops, cut to a thickness of ¾-inch to 1-inch (1.9-cm to 2.5-cm). A bone-in steak or chop can be cooked the same way, but you will need to add about 2 minutes more cooking time per side. Always season the meat with a little salt and freshly ground black pepper on both sides before cooking. To jazz up any of these techniques, you can add a pat of garlic and herb butter to the meat right before serving, or make a wine reduction in the pan for a sauce.

PAN-GRILLED STEAK OR CHOP
Use a cast iron grill pan with a heavy ridged bottom. Lightly oil the pan and preheat it over medium-high heat. When it is hot, but not smoking, add the seasoned steak or chop. Cook for 5 minutes per side, flipping (with tongs, not a fork) only once, for medium-rare. Shorten or lengthen the cooking time for rare or well done. Remove from the heat and let the meat sit on a platter under a loose foil tent for about 3 minutes before serving.

BROILED STEAK OR CHOP
Preheat broiler. Set oven rack approximately 6 inches (15.2 cm) below broiler.

Lightly oil a broiler pan and place the seasoned steaks or chops on it. Place under the broiler so that the meat is approximately 5 inches (12.7 cm) below the heat. Broil for about 4 to 5 minutes per side, turning only once. Watch closely as some broilers can be very fast. Remove from the heat and let the meat sit on a platter under a loose foil tent for about 3 minutes before serving.

Basic Pan-Grilled or
Broiled Steaks and Chops (continued)

TO MAKE A GARLIC & HERB BUTTER

Mix 4 tablespoons (56 g) of softened butter with 2 finely minced garlic cloves, 2 tablespoons (8 g) of mixed finely chopped fresh herbs of your choice such as flat leaf parsley, chives, tarragon, basil, marjoram, cilantro or rosemary; add salt and freshly ground black pepper to taste. Chill. Place a teaspoon of the butter on top of each steak or chop right before serving.

TO MAKE A WINE REDUCTION

This is something you can do if you have cooked the steak or chop in a skillet.

After transferring the cooked steak or chop from the skillet to a platter and covering with a loose foil tent, add 2 tablespoons (20 g) minced shallot to the hot skillet and cook until tender and lightly browned (about 2 minutes, stirring). Add in 1 cup (235 ml) red wine and bring it to a boil, whisking constantly to loosen any brown bits from the bottom of the pan, and cook until the wine is reduced by half. Whisk in 3 tablespoons (42 g) of cold butter. Season with salt and freshly ground black pepper. Spoon a little over the steak as you serve it.

Per Serving: Calories will vary (sirloin steak is 474) • GL 0 • Glycals 0
With a green salad: Calories 507 • GL 0 • Glycals 1
❢ Add a glass of red wine: Calories 606 • GL 0 • Glycals 1

Chicken Tenders Provençale

Satisfying and economical, chicken is perhaps the most versatile low-glycal food. From start to finish, you can have this savory low-glycal dish on the table in 30 minutes and the meat will be surrounded by a savory sauce of tomatoes, garlic, thyme and wine—classic Provençale ingredients.

The cut of chicken referred to as "tenders" is more flavorful and juicy than the breast—perfect for this meal.

YIELD: 4 SERVINGS

2 lb (910 g) chicken tenders

3 tbsp (45 ml) olive oil

8 plum tomatoes, halved lengthwise

4 garlic cloves, peeled and halved

2 tsp (2 g) dried thyme, crushed

½ cup (120 ml) white wine

Salt and freshly ground pepper

Preheat oven to 400°F (200°C). Heat the oil in a large cast iron skillet. When it is hot, but not smoking, add the chicken. Cook until browned on all sides; remove from skillet and set on a plate.

Add the tomatoes, garlic, thyme and wine to the pan. Season with a little salt and pepper. Cook over medium-high heat for a minute or two or until the tomatoes begin to get soft. Add the chicken (and any juices that have formed on the plate) to the skillet and cover with a tight-fitting lid. Lower the heat and cook at a low simmer for 20 minutes, or until the chicken is completely cooked. Serve immediately.

Per Serving: Calories 484 • GL 1 • Glycals 4
With serving of spinach: Calories 512 • GL 1 • Glycals 7
❢ Add a glass of white wine: Calories 611 • GL 1 • Glycals 9

Chicken with White Wine

On the Low-Glycal Diet, you can enjoy wine with dinner, and you can cook with wine, too! This dish is another example of a chicken recipe that's greater than the sum of its parts. Pan-browned pieces of chicken are topped with a sauce of shallots, rosemary and wine that's quickly made in the same skillet you cooked the chicken in. Good any time of year, this recipe is particularly appealing during the cold weather months. If you are not cooking for a crowd, you'll find the extra chicken can be portioned and stored in the freezer for a meal that, once defrosted, is ready to go in minutes.

YIELD: 6 SERVINGS

3½ lb (1.6 kg) chicken parts, bone-in, skin on

Salt and freshly ground black pepper

1 tbsp (15 ml) olive oil

2 shallots, sliced (approx. 3 tbsp [30 g])

1 tbsp (1.7 g) chopped fresh rosemary

½ cup (120 ml) dry white wine

½ cup (120 ml) chicken stock or broth

Preheat oven to 450°F (230°C). Rinse the chicken under cold running water and pat dry with a paper towel. Season with salt and pepper. Place the oil in a large ovenproof skillet (cast iron is best), set over medium-high heat. As soon as the oil is hot, but not smoking, add some of the chicken to the pan and brown quickly on both sides. Work in small batches (this will allow the skin to get a deep golden-brown color without entirely cooking the chicken), transferring the browned chicken pieces to a plate as you go.

When all the pieces have been browned, return the chicken to the pan, placing it skin-side up, and sprinkle the shallots and rosemary over it. Place in the oven, uncovered, and roast for approximately 20 minutes, or until the juices run clear when you cut into a piece. Remove the skillet from the oven and, using tongs, transfer the cooked chicken to a serving platter; cover with foil to keep hot.

Place the skillet over medium-high heat. Add the wine and broth to the pan and bring to a boil, scraping up the brown bits on the bottom of the pan with a whisk. Simmer over medium-low until reduced by half. Strain the sauce into a pitcher; pour it over the cooked chicken pieces. Serve immediately.

Per Serving: Calories 396 • GL 0 • Glycals 1
With green beans, small salad and bleu cheese dressing:
Calories 447 • GL 1 • Glycals 3
❢ Add a glass of white wine: Calories 546 • GL 1 • Glycals 4

Herbed Whole Roasted Chicken

On its own, roasted chicken is a zero GL/zero glycal food; add a green vegetable and a salad and you have a low-glycal dinner (add potatoes, and it becomes high-glycal). This dish is ideal for a casual dinner with friends because you're free to socialize while the chicken cooks and fills the kitchen with a mouth-watering aroma. Only a few ingredients are needed but, as you'll see, the results are greater than the sum of its parts: a crispy flavorful skin and super-moist meat. Maybe that's why many famous chefs have cited whole roasted chicken as a go-to favorite. It's bound to become one of yours, too.

Save the carcass for chicken stock. Leftover meat can be used in a chicken salad.

YIELD: 4–6 SERVINGS

---

1 whole chicken, 4 lb (1.8 kg)

1 onion, peeled and halved

½ lemon

6 garlic cloves, peeled and halved

1 tbsp (15 ml) olive oil

1 tsp salt

Freshly ground pepper

1 tsp each (dried): thyme, rosemary, and sage

Preheat oven to 450°F (230°C). Remove and discard any excess fat from the inside of the chicken; remove the neck, heart and liver and freeze for use in chicken stock or discard. Rinse the chicken inside and out under cold running water. Set on paper towels, pat dry and transfer to the roasting pan, breast-side up. To prevent them from burning, twist and tuck the wing tips under the chicken.

Place the onion, lemon and garlic in the body cavity. Drizzle the olive oil over the bird and, with your hands, rub it on evenly. Clean your hands; sprinkle the salt and pepper over the chicken. Working with one dried herb at a time, place the measured amount in the palm of your hand and rub your palms together over the chicken to crush the herbs and release more of their flavors.

Place the chicken in the oven and roast for 1 hour. If your oven is "uneven" you will need to rotate the pan every 20 minutes to get an even browning of the skin.

Remove the roasting pan from the oven and transfer the chicken to a platter. Allow the chicken to rest under a loose foil tent for 10 minutes before carving.

During this time, pour the roasting pan juices into a small saucepan over medium-high heat. Add ¼ cup (60 ml) water and scrape up any brown bits from the bottom of the pan. Bring the mixture to a boil, immediately reduce to a simmer, and let cook for 2 minutes.

Carve the chicken into serving pieces; pour the reduced cooking juices over the slices and serve.

Per Serving: Calories 357 • GL 0 • Glycals 0
With green beans: Calories 394 • GL 1 • Glycals 3
❢ Add a glass of wine: Calories 493 • GL 1 • Glycals 3

Parmesan Chicken Breasts

Here's a dish that's so quickly and easily prepared, you can pull it off even after a long day at the office. Dredging the chicken in flour or bread crumbs or cornmeal—which may be how you are accustomed to doing it—would make this a high-glycal dish but the dredge of Parmesan cheese does not. And, it adds tremendous flavor!

YIELD: 2 SERVINGS

2 chicken breasts, boneless, skinless

2 eggs, beaten

¼ cup (25 g) freshly grated Parmesan cheese

½ tsp dried oregano, crushed

2 tbsp (30 ml) olive oil

Preheat oven to 375°F (190°C). Dip the chicken breasts in the beaten eggs, then in the Parmesan cheese. Sprinkle the dried oregano over the top of the chicken. Place on a lightly oiled baking pan and bake for 20 to 30 minutes, or until the chicken is completely cooked.

Remove from oven and serve.

Per Serving: Calories 598 • GL 0 • Glycals 0
With salad: Calories 657 • GL • Glycals 1
❢ Add a glass of red wine: Calories 759 • GL 0 • Glycals 1

Parmesan Pork Chops

Chops make a great low-glycal choice for a weeknight dinner because they cook quickly—once you have all the ingredients at hand, they will be ready to eat in under 15 minutes. A flour dredge would make this dish high-glycal, whereas the Parmesan keeps it low-glycal and adds a melt-in-your-mouth crust that keeps the pork extra juicy. Pork's flavor makes it a good-for-all-seasons main course that can be complemented by seasonal vegetables or fruits. This recipe is especially appealing during the fall and winter.

YIELD: 2 SERVINGS

2 pork chops, boneless*
(approx. 1" [2.5-cm] thick)

2 eggs, beaten

¼ cup (25 g) freshly grated
Parmesan cheese

2 tbsp (30 ml) olive oil

Preheat oven to 375°F (190°C). Dip the pork chops in the beaten eggs, and then in the Parmesan cheese, coating both sides equally. Set aside on a platter.

Add the olive oil to a skillet set over medium-high heat. When the oil is hot, but not smoking, add the chops to the pan and lower the heat to medium. Set a timer and cook the chops for 4 minutes per side (or until golden brown), turning only once. Do *not* move the chops around the pan.

Transfer the chops to an oven-proof dish and finish in the oven for 5 minutes, or until desired doneness. Remove from oven and allow to sit for 3 minutes before serving.

*Note: Bone-in chops will require another minute per side in the skillet, and a couple of minutes longer in the oven.

Per Serving: Calories 631 • GL 0 • Glycals 0
With Brussels sprouts: Calories 700 • GL 1 • Glycals 4
❢ Add a glass of red or white wine: Calories 802 • GL 1 • Glycals 5

Baked Pork Spare Ribs

Here's a quickly prepared, economical dish that is especially satisfying during cooler weather. Assembly takes 15 minutes, max; then, pop this meal-in-one dish in the oven for an hour. Rich-tasting because of the rendered fat, pork spare ribs are a low-glycal food.

YIELD: 4 SERVINGS

4 lb (1.8 kg) pork spare ribs

Salt and freshly ground black pepper

2 onions, quartered

2 green apples, quartered

½ head red cabbage, cored, halved and sliced into ¼" (6-mm) sections

1 tbsp (8 g) grated fresh ginger

1 tbsp (15 ml) olive oil

Preheat oven to 350°F (180°C). Lightly oil a 9 x 12-inch (23 x 30.5-cm) baking pan. Season the spare ribs with a little salt and pepper and place in pan. Distribute the onions and apples evenly over the pork. Tuck bunches of the red cabbage into any spaces between the pork (do not spread cabbage out in a thin layer). Mix the ginger with the olive oil and spoon it over the ingredients. Bake in preheated oven for 1 hour. Serve hot.

Per Serving: Calories 508 • GL 2 • Glycals 8
🍷 Add a glass of wine: Calories 610 • GL 2 • Glycals 10

Mustard Glazed Pork Tenderloin

Pork tenderloin is a tender, flavorful, lean cut that can be enhanced with a variety of treatments. Here, a quick marinade featuring Dijon mustard, soy sauce and garlic adds a tangy complement to each juicy bite. As with all cuts of pork, tenderloin is a zero GL food. It is also a terrific source of vitamin B6 and other important nutrients.

YIELD: 4 SERVINGS

1½ lb (680 g) pork tenderloin

2 tbsp (28 g) Dijon mustard

2 tbsp (30 ml) olive oil

1 tbsp (15 ml) soy sauce

1 garlic clove, pressed

¼ tsp freshly ground pepper

Preheat your broiler. Score the tenderloin, making ¼ inch (6 mm) deep cuts diagonally every 2 inches (5.1 cm). Set in the boiler pan.

In a bowl, whisk together the mustard, oil, soy sauce, garlic and pepper. Brush half the marinade on the pork and let it stand 10 minutes.

Place the tenderloin 4 inches (10.2 cm) below the broiler and cook for 8 minutes. Quickly turn the roast over and brush with remaining marinade. Return to the broiler for another 8 to 10 minutes. Let it rest on a platter under a loose foil tent for a few minutes before slicing.

Per Serving: Calories 492 • GL 0 • Glycals 0
With spinach: Calories 521 • GL 1 • Glycals 4
❣ Add a glass of red wine: Calories 623 • GL 1 • Glycals 5

Parmesan Honey Roast Pork Tenderloin

Can also be served for lunch (green)

Talk about easy! With very little effort on your part this recipe makes a juicy roast that develops a sticky, flavorful "crust" as it cooks that will awe your dinner guests. Or, put it on the menu for a Sunday dinner for two and enjoy the leftovers during the week. The ingredient that makes this dish medium-glycal after 6:00 p.m. is the honey. If you eliminated it, the dish would be low-glycal for lunch or dinner.

YIELD: 6 SERVINGS

---

1 (2 lb [910 g]) pork loin roast, boneless

2 tbsp (30 ml) olive oil

Salt and pepper

2 tbsp (40 g) honey

2 tbsp (30 ml) soy sauce

2 tbsp (6.6 g) dried rosemary

2 tbsp (20 g) finely minced garlic

⅓ cup (33 g) grated Parmesan cheese

Preheat oven to 450°F (230°C). Place the roast in a baking pan. Season evenly on all sides with salt and pepper.

In a bowl, whisk together the olive oil, honey and soy sauce. In your palms, crush and rub the rosemary over the bowl; add the garlic and Parmesan cheese and mix well.

Using a spoon and your fingers, coat the roast evenly with the mixture.

Bake for 30 to 40 minutes, depending on your preference for doneness (or until a meat thermometer reads 160°F [71°C]).

Let the roast sit under a loose foil tent for 5 minutes before slicing.

FOR LUNCH (green), on a bed of greens
Per Serving: Calories 703 • GL 2 • Glycals 12

FOR DINNER (yellow), with 5 spears steamed asparagus
Per Serving: Calories 718 • GL 2 • Glycals 15
🍷 Add a glass of red wine: Calories 820 • GL 2 • Glycals 17

Leeks, Peas & Mushrooms with Grilled Italian Sausage Over Pasta

Thank goodness for the flexibility of the Low-Glycal Diet! You can enjoy this dish during Step 2 (when you are allowed one high-glycal meal a week) and during Step 3 (when you can have a whole day every week of high-glycal meals!). The prep is a bit time-consuming but if you have friends who like to cook with you before sitting down to enjoy a special meal, this recipe fits the bill.

The pasta is the ingredient that makes this dish high-glycal.

YIELD: 6 SERVINGS

2 cups (210 g) thinly sliced leeks (white and pale green parts only)

1½ cups (350 ml) dry white vermouth (or white wine)

4 tbsp (56 g) butter, cut into ½" (1.3-cm) cubes

3 tbsp (45 g) cream

Salt and freshly ground black pepper

3 tbsp (45 ml) olive oil

1 lb (455 g) mushrooms (crimini, small portobello, shiitake, button), cut into wedges

¼ cup (50 g) sliced shallots

1 (10-oz [280-g]) package frozen peas, thawed

2 tbsp (8 g) chopped fresh flat leaf parsley, divided

2 tsp (1.5 g) chopped fresh thyme

4 tbsp (20 g) grated Parmesan cheese

1½ lb (680 g) sweet Italian sausage, large links, grilled; sliced on the diagonal into 2" (5 cm) pieces

1 lb (455 g) pasta, cooked al dente

Place the leeks and vermouth in a saucepan over high heat and bring to a boil; lower the heat and cook at a simmer until the liquid is reduced to approximately ⅓ cup (78 ml). Remove the pan from the heat and stir in the butter, a few pieces at a time. Add the cream, and return the pot to very low heat, whisking to prevent scorching, and cook for 1 minute. Season with salt and pepper and remove from the heat.

Heat the olive oil in a large skillet set over medium-high heat. Add the mushrooms and sauté for 5 minutes. Stir in the shallots, 1 tablespoon (4 g) of the parsley and all of the thyme. Continue cooking until the mushrooms are very tender, about 5 minutes more. Add the peas; toss well. Remove from the heat and add the leek mixture. Set aside.

Place the drained cooked pasta in a large shallow serving bowl. Pour the leek, mushroom and pea mixture over the pasta and add the remaining fresh parsley. Toss to distribute evenly. Sprinkle the Parmesan cheese over all and serve with grilled Italian sausages.

Per Serving: Calories 712 • GL 20 • Glycals 131
Add a glass of wine: Calories 811 • GL 20 • Glycals 149

Beef Provençale Style

An old-fashioned traditional French recipe from the Provence area, this dish calls for simple ingredients—starring tomatoes, thyme and olives—that combine with the juices from the beef to yield a richly flavored low-glycal meal.

To peel a tomato: dip it into a pot of boiling water; remove immediately and set to cool on a plate. The skin will wrinkle slightly and lift off easily.

YIELD: 6 SERVINGS

4 tbsp (60 ml) olive oil

2 onions, peeled, halved and sliced from stem to root end

4 cups (720 g) chopped ripe tomatoes (peeled and seeded)

1 tsp dried thyme, crushed

½ bay leaf

1 garlic clove, thinly sliced

2 tbsp (8 g) chopped fresh flat leaf parsley

2 lb (910 g) of stew beef (tenderloin or whatever your butcher recommends, cut in 1" [2.5-cm] cubes)

Salt and freshly ground black pepper

¾ cup (75 g) Kalamata olives, rough chopped

Heat the oil in a heavy-bottomed pot set over medium heat and when it is hot but not smoking add the onion and cook, stirring occasionally with a wooden spoon, until the onions are a light golden color. Add the tomatoes, thyme, bay leaf, garlic and parsley. Continue cooking the mixture for 5 minutes, stirring occasionally. Add the beef and season with a little salt and pepper. Add the olives. Stir once, cover with a tight fitting lid and reduce the heat to the *lowest* setting. Cook for approximately 15 minutes more. Turn off the heat and let the covered pot sit for 20 minutes. Serve with a crisp green salad.

Per Serving: Calories 556 • GL 1 • Glycals 6
🍷 Add a glass of red wine: Calories 658 • GL 2 • Glycals 7

Open-Face Lamb Burger with Yogurt Sauce

Can also be served for lunch (yellow)

If you like lamb, you'll love this recipe. Juicy, flavorful burgers, grilled sourdough bread, mixed baby salad greens and a tangy, garlicky yogurt sauce—yum. It's a meal-in-one-dish, and will become an instant favorite for a casual weekend dinner with friends. By the way, if you're "off" bread, leave it out; you'll still end up with a fabulous dish.

YIELD: 4 SERVINGS

FOR THE YOGURT SAUCE

1 cup (230 g) plain yogurt (before spooning yogurt out of the carton, pour off any liquid on top)

1 cup (100 g) loosely packed whole fresh mint leaves plus 2 tbsp (12 g) minced

1 tsp fresh lemon juice

1 garlic clove, halved lengthwise

FOR THE LAMB BURGERS

1½ lbs (680 g) ground lamb (not lean; shoulder cut is good)

⅓ cup (20 g) minced fresh flat leaf parsley

¼ cup (40 g) minced onion

Salt and freshly ground black pepper

Pinch (⅛ tsp) ground allspice

4 thick (½" [1.3-cm]) slices sourdough bread (from a crusty loaf)

2 tbsp (30 ml) plus 1 tsp olive oil

3 cups (345 g) mixed baby salad greens

To make the Yogurt Sauce whisk together yogurt, minced mint, lemon juice and salt to taste. Mince ½ of the garlic clove and whisk into yogurt sauce.

To make the Lamb Patties mix lamb, parsley, onion, salt, pepper and allspice in a bowl until just combined (use your hands and do not overwork mixture or patties will be tough). Form into 4 patties.

Preheat the grill; grill the bread.

Brush both sides of the bread slices with oil (2 tablespoons [30 ml] total for all) and grill, turning once, until golden on both sides, 1 to 2 minutes total. Rub 1 side of each piece of toast with the cut side of remaining garlic clove and season with a pinch of salt.

Grill patties on a hot lightly oiled grill rack, turning over once, until nicely browned on the outside but still slightly pink in center (5 to 7 minutes total depending on the grill).

Toss together the baby salad greens with the whole mint leaves, the remaining teaspoon of olive oil and salt and pepper to taste.

Place the lamb burgers on the grilled bread, arrange a portion of greens around each and spoon a little yogurt sauce over all. Place extra yogurt sauce in a small pitcher on the table.

Note: If you prefer to cook indoors, the burgers can be cooked in a hot lightly oiled cast iron pan (ridged is best) over moderately high heat, or under the broiler, turning over once.

Per Serving: Calories 621 • GL 7 • Glycals 40
🍷 Add a glass of wine: Calories 723 • GL 7 • Glycals 40
Note: Only the bread makes this a high-glycal dish.

Grilled Flank Steak

Flank steak is extremely lean so it really should be marinated or it will be dry. Cook this under the broiler or over a bed of hot charcoals on an outdoor grill. This cut has a nice chewy texture, which, along with the varied ways you can prepare it and its zero GL/glycal profile, makes it a go-to choice in your low-glycal meal plan. Any leftover slices can be used in a steak and avocado wrap for lunch.

YIELD: 2 SERVINGS

1 lb (455 g) flank steak, scored lightly on both sides

Freshly ground black pepper

¼ cup (59 ml) olive oil

3 tbsp (45 ml) fresh lemon juice

2 tbsp (30 ml) soy sauce

2 garlic cloves, minced

Rub both sides of the steak with pepper. In a shallow dish just large enough to hold the steak, whisk together the oil, lemon juice, soy sauce and garlic. Add the steak, coating both sides well with the marinade. Let the steak marinate, turning it once, for 20 minutes.

Remove the steak from the marinade, and grill it on an oiled rack over glowing coals, 5 minutes per side, brushing it occasionally with some of the marinade and turning it only once, for medium-rare meat. Or, broil the steak under a preheated broiler about 4 inches (10.2 cm) from the heat, turning it once, for 5 minutes per side for medium-rare meat. Discard marinade. Transfer the steak to a warm platter. Let it stand for 5 minutes under a loose foil tent. Slice the steak thinly across the grain and serve.

Per Serving: Calories 781 • GL 0 • Glycals 2
❢ Add a glass of red wine, small spinach salad with bleu cheese dressing: Calories 1076 • GL 1 • Glycals 9

Grilled Rib-Eye Steak

If you are a beef steak lover, rejoice! Your favorite food is a zero GL/glycal food. The rib-eye cut has a tremendously rich flavor and tender juicy texture (think: prime rib). You don't need to marinate it or do anything other than season it with a little salt and pepper to enhance its flavors. You certainly can cook the steak on an outdoor grill but it's just as good cooked on top of the stove in a high-quality grill pan. The best grill pans are cast iron with a heavy ridged bottom (mine, 8-inch [20.3-cm] diameter, weighs 6 pounds [2.72 kg]!).

YIELD: 4 SERVINGS

2 (1 lb [455 g]) boneless rib-eye steaks, at room temperature

Salt and freshly ground black pepper, to taste

Light a grill or, if cooking indoors, preheat a grilling pan over medium-high heat. Season the steaks with salt and pepper. When the grill or grilling pan is hot, place the steaks on the surface and set a timer for 5 minutes. Do not move the steaks while they cook, and do not press on them! Using tongs (not a fork), turn the steaks over and cook for another 5 minutes. This should yield a medium-rare steak. If you like medium or well done, add another 1 to 2 minutes of cooking time per side.

Transfer the steaks to a cutting board, cover with a loose foil tent and let them rest for 5 minutes. Cut the steaks across the grain into thick slices and serve.

Note: If you are using a gas grill, you will need to allow 1 to 2 minutes more per side than you would over a charcoal fire. If you are cooking on a traditional grill over hardwood charcoals, set the grilling surface about 6 inches (15.2 cm) above the hot coals.

Per Serving: Calories 686 • GL 0 • Glycals 0
With a small Caesar Salad: Calories 858 • GL 0 • Glycals 1
🍷 Add a glass of red wine: Calories 960 • GL 0 • Glycals 2

Marinated Grilled Sirloin Steak

A good sirloin steak needs no adornment but this marinade brings its juicy flavor to another level of wow, this is good! The steak can be marinated for up to a day in advance. Low-glycal? Or course—all meat is. And, it's high in B vitamins.

YIELD: 2 SERVINGS

¾ lb (340 g) New York-cut sirloin steak, about 1" (2.5-cm) thick

3 tbsp (45 ml) balsamic vinegar

1 tbsp (15 ml) olive oil

2 garlic cloves, minced

½ tsp dried thyme, crushed

Salt and freshly ground pepper

In a large, sealable plastic bag, combine the vinegar, oil, garlic and thyme. Add the steak, making sure to coat both sides with the marinade. Press out any air in the bag and seal it tightly. Place on a plate (in case of leaks) and refrigerate for at least 4 hours, preferably overnight. Allow the steak to come to room temperature before grilling.

Oil and preheat the grill or skillet. Place the steak on the hot grill or skillet over medium-high heat, brushing the topside of the steak with marinade. Cook one side for 4 minutes; using tongs, flip the steak and brush with a little marinade. Cook the other side for 4 to 5 minutes for medium-rare, a minute or two longer for medium. (Discard leftover marinade.)

Transfer the cooked steak to a cutting board. Allow to rest for 5 minutes. Serve.

Per Serving: Calories 510 • GL 0 • Glycals 0
With a small salad: Per Serving: Calories 545 • GL 1 • Glycals 4
❢ Add a glass of red wine: Calories 647 • GL 1 • Glycals 5

Wine-Braised Beef Short Ribs

Braising means cooking "low and slow" in a liquid—in this case, a savory mixture of root vegetables, herbs and red wine. Preparing this dish before it goes in the oven will take some time but once it goes in, you can walk away for 2 hours. A perfect dinner on a cold winter's day. The beef (of course) is low-glycal; to keep the dish that way do not increase the carrots unless you are planning a medium- or high-glycal meal.

YIELD: 4 SERVINGS

3 lb (1.36 kg) bone-in beef short ribs (have the butcher cut them crosswise into 2″ [5.1-cm] pieces)

Salt and freshly ground black pepper

3 tbsp (45 ml) olive oil

2 onions, chopped

2 carrots, chopped

2 celery stalks, chopped

1 tbsp (15 g) tomato paste

4 cups (946 ml) dry red wine (Cabernet Sauvignon is a good choice)

1 bay leaf

2 tsp (2.8 g) dried thyme

1 garlic head, halved crosswise (unpeeled)

4 cups (946 ml) beef stock

Preheat oven to 350°F (180°C). Season the beef with salt and pepper. Heat the oil in a large Dutch oven over medium-high heat until very hot but not smoking; add half the ribs and brown on all sides (about 6 minutes total); you will have to work in 2 batches unless the Dutch oven is very large. When done, transfer the ribs to a plate. Save 3 tablespoons (45 ml) of drippings from the pot, and discard the rest.

Add the onions, carrots and celery to the pot and cook, stirring often, until the onions are browned, about 5 minutes. Stir in the tomato paste, add the wine and return the short ribs (with any juices that have accumulated on the plate) to the pot. Bring to a simmer and cook over low heat, partially covered, for 15 to 20 minutes or until the wine is reduced by half.

Add all the herbs and garlic. Stir in the stock. Return to a simmer, cover tightly and transfer to the oven. Cook for 2 hours.

Using tongs, transfer the short ribs to a platter and cover with a loose foil tent. Strain the cooking liquid into wide bowl, and skim the fat from the surface; pour the skimmed sauce into a pitcher. Serve in shallow bowls with a portion of sauce over each.

For a red meal treat, serve with mashed potatoes.

Per Serving: Calories 527 • GL 1 • Glycals 5
❢ Add a glass of red wine: Calories 629 • GL 1 • Glycals 6
With mashed potatoes: Calories 737 • GL 18 • Glycals 124

Whole Roasted Sirloin

This cut of beef is expensive—but so worth it! Intensely flavored, juicy, and with a satisfyingly chewy yet tender texture, when you need a main course for a special occasion like a holiday party, this roast fits the bill. Before you head out to buy it, however, call to make sure one is available; it may have to be cut for you. Your butcher won't mind—the sirloin roast is considered a connoisseur's favorite.

You can start the prep for this dish a day in advance because the "dry rub," which intensifies the meat's flavor and juiciness, can be applied up to 24 hours before roasting—another plus when you're hosting a crowd. By the way, the fresh thyme is a must.

YIELD: 6–8 SERVINGS

THE ROAST

1 tbsp (18 g) kosher salt

½ tsp coarse ground black pepper

¼ tsp dry mustard

1 garlic clove, finely minced

1½ tbsp (3.6 g) fresh thyme, coarsely chopped

1 (5 lb [2.26 kg]) sirloin roast

THE SAUCE

2 cups (475 ml) red wine

4 cups (946 ml) beef stock

2 tbsp (4.8 g) fresh thyme, finely chopped

1 pinch kosher salt

1 tsp butter

In a small bowl, mix the salt, pepper, mustard, garlic and thyme together well. Place the roast on a platter and, using your hands, generously season it with the mixture, patting it onto all sides. Cover with plastic wrap and refrigerate for up to 24 hours, or until you are ready to cook it.

Preheat oven temperature to 450°F (230°C). Set the roast on a roasting rack in a roasting pan, fat-side up. If any of the dry rub is left behind on the platter, add it to the top of the roast. Place the roast in the hot oven and cook for approximately 1 hour or until the meat reaches an internal temperature of 125°F (51°C) (for medium-rare). Remove the pan from oven and let sit for a minute or so before transferring the roast (using tongs, not forks) to a carving platter. Cover with a loose foil tent and let the roast rest for 10 minutes before carving.

While the meat rests, make the sauce: Skim off the fat in the roasting pan; place the pan over medium-high heat and when it's hot add the red wine. Using a wooden spoon, stir gently and loosen any browned bits on the bottom of the pan. When the wine has been reduced by half, add the stock and continue to cook, stirring, until the mixture is reduced by half again. Whisk in the thyme, salt and butter; pour into a small pitcher.

Carve roast to desired thickness and serve with the sauce on the side.

Note: Any leftovers make a delicious treat for a low-glycal lunch. Serve on a bed of mesclun greens with crumbled bleu cheese.

Per Serving: Calories 314 • GL 0 • Glycals 0
❗ Add a glass of red wine: Calories 416 • GL 0 • Glycals 0
With steamed spinach: Calories 444 • GL 1 • Glycals 3
For red meal, add roasted root vegetables and mashed potatoes!

Pot Roast

Rump roast is an inexpensive cut that is greatly enhanced by the technique of searing in hot oil followed by a slow finish in a savory broth. Enriched by the root vegetables, the broth becomes a gravy for the sliced roast. This recipe serves a crowd, or provides leftovers for low-glycal lunches.

Note: This is a green (low-glycal) meal at lunch, so keep that in mind for a Sunday dinner.

YIELD: 6 SERVINGS

---

4 tbsp (60 ml) olive oil, divided

6 onions, peeled

2 garlic cloves, peeled

1 (4 lb [1.8 kg]) boneless rump roast

Salt and freshly ground black pepper

5 cups (1.18 L) beef stock

1 cup (235 ml) apple cider

1 tsp dried thyme, crushed

1 bay leaf

1 tbsp (15 g) tomato paste

6 carrots or parsnips, scrubbed

Preheat oven to 350°F (180°C). Heat 2 tablespoons (30 ml) of the oil in a large Dutch oven set over medium heat and when it is hot, but not smoking, add the whole onions and garlic. Sear the onions until browned (they will not be tender). Remove the pot from the heat; using a slotted spoon, remove the onions from the pot and set aside. Remove the garlic; mash and set aside in a small bowl.

Season the roast generously with salt and pepper.

Return the Dutch oven to medium-high heat, and add the remaining 2 tablespoons (30 ml) of oil. When the oil is hot, add the roast and brown it on all sides, turning with tongs only as each side is browned. Add the beef stock, cider, thyme, bay leaf, tomato paste and mashed garlic to the pot. Bring to a boil, cover and place the Dutch oven in the preheated oven. Bake for 90 minutes. Add the carrots or parsnips, and seared onions to the pot. Cover and continue to cook in the oven for another 40 minutes or until the meat and vegetables are completely tender.

To serve, remove the roast to a platter, and allow to sit for at least 5 minutes before carving. Arrange the vegetables on a serving platter. Ladle the cooking liquid over the meat and vegetables as each plate is served.

Per Serving: Calories 395 • GL 6 • Glycals 23
❢ Add a glass of red wine: Calories 497 • GL 6 • Glycals 29
Caution: Wine makes this meal red (high-glycal)
Note: Without parsnips but with wine, this is a
green (low-glycal) dinner:
Calories 472 • GL 2 • Glycals 10

Veal Cutlets with Basil

Veal is low-glycal, like all meat, but it is often dredged in flour, which changes it to a high-glycal food. Here, a simple preparation yields elegant results. Serve with a steamed green vegetable (spinach or Swiss chard goes well with this) and a salad and you have a satisfying and tasty low-glycal dinner.

YIELD: 4 SERVINGS

4 veal cutlets

Salt and freshly ground black pepper

½ cup (120 ml) olive oil

8 tbsp (112 g) butter (1 stick), softened

3 tbsp (7.5 g) finely minced fresh basil

Cook the cutlets in a dry skillet set over medium-high heat until browned, about 3 minutes per side. Season with salt and pepper and set aside on a platter under a loose foil tent.

Using a whisk or hand-held mixer, combine the oil and butter to form a smooth paste. Add the basil.

Top each cutlet with 1 tablespoon (15 g) of the basil butter, and serve immediately.

Per Serving: Calories 659 • GL 0 • Glycals 0
❢ Add a glass of wine: Calories 758 • GL 0 • Glycals 0

Cod Provençale

Cod is a fish that is as adaptable to diverse preparations and flavors as chicken. It has a beautifully flakey white meat and, on its own, a sweet nutty flavor. No wonder it is one of the most popular seafoods in America, and around the world. Like all seafood, cod is low-glycal—as long as you don't dredge it in flour or breadcrumbs or cornmeal. Here, it's cooked with the classic Provençale ingredients of tomatoes, olives and basil, yielding a savory sauce that complements the fish.

YIELD: 4 SERVINGS

2 tbsp (30 ml) olive oil

2 tbsp (28 g) butter

⅔ cup (106 g) chopped onion

1 garlic clove, minced

2 lb (910 g) cod fillets

8 plum tomatoes, peeled, seeded and chopped

8 Kalamata olives, pitted and rough chopped

½ tsp chopped fresh thyme

1 tbsp (2.5 g) chopped fresh basil

Place the oil and butter in a large, heavy skillet set over medium heat. Add the onion and cook, stirring occasionally, until the onions become tender. Add the garlic and cook until the garlic is fragrant but not browned. Remove the onions and garlic from the pan, and set aside. Return the pan to the heat, and when it is hot, but not smoking, add the cod fillets and cook for about 1 minute.

Return the onions and garlic to the pan with the fish. Add the tomatoes, olives and thyme, sprinkling over and around the fish. Turn the heat to medium-low, cover the skillet with a tight-fitting lid and cook for about 3 to 4 minutes more, or until the fish is cooked and the onions are tender.

Place a fillet on each plate, and spoon the onions, garlic and tomato mix over the fish, using all the juices that form in the pan. Sprinkle some fresh basil over each and serve immediately.

Per Serving: Calories 238 • GL 1 • Glycals 3
With a green salad: Calories 296 • GL 1 • Glycals 4
❢ Add a glass of white wine: Calories 395 • GL 1 • Glycals 5

Oven-Baked Fish Chowder

Can also be served for Lunch

This is the easiest chowder you'll ever make: Put the ingredients in a Dutch oven, bake for an hour and enjoy a richly flavored chock-full-of-fish chowder! And it's just as good made with water if you don't have fish stock on hand. Most restaurant or canned chowders are high-glycal because they contain potatoes—so don't add them to this recipe unless you want to create a high-glycal dish.

YIELD: 6 SERVINGS

2 lb (910 g) cod, haddock, hake or any firm white fish fillets

1½ cups (180 g) diced celery

1½ cups (240 g) diced onion

1 bay leaf

1 tsp salt

¼ tsp freshly ground black pepper

½ cup (120 ml) dry white wine

4 tbsp (55 g) butter

2 cups (475 ml) boiling water or fish stock

1 cup (235 ml) milk

2 tsp (2.6 g) chopped fresh parsley

Preheat oven to 375°F (190°C). Rub your fingertips along the fish to feel for bones, and remove any with tweezers. Place the fish fillets, whole, in a 4 quart (3.78 L) Dutch oven or other ovenproof casserole that can be transferred later to the top of the stove. *Do not cut up the fish*; it will flake into bite-size pieces as it cooks. Add all the remaining ingredients except the milk and parsley. Cover the pot and bake for 1 hour.

Transfer the Dutch oven to the top of the stove, over low heat. Slowly stir in the milk. Let it sit over low heat for 5 to 10 minutes. Add the fresh parsley and serve immediately.

Per Serving: Calories 207 • GL 1 • Glycals 2
🍷 Add a glass of white wine: Calories 306 • GL 1 • Glycals 3

Seafood Chowder

Can also be served for lunch

This chowder of clams, scallops, shrimp and fish gets better with age, so make the full recipe even if you're not feeding a crowd. The seafood is low-glycal; if you add potatoes this chowder becomes high-glycal.

YIELD: 6 SERVINGS

---

24 live quahogs (hard-shell clams)

1 cup (235 ml) water

½ cup (120 ml) dry white wine

4 tbsp (55 g) butter (½ a stick)

1½ cups (240 g) chopped onion

¾ cup (75 g) chopped celery

2 cups (475 ml) fish stock

1 bay leaf

½ tsp chopped fresh thyme

½ lb (225 g) shucked scallops

½ lb (225 g) medium shrimp (wild), shell left on tail, deveined

½ lb (225 g) fish cut in 1″ (2.5-cm) cubes (monkfish, cod, haddock or other firm white fish)

3 cups (705 ml) milk

Salt and white pepper, to taste

1 tbsp (4 g) chopped fresh flat leaf parsley

Scrub the quahog shells under cold running water to remove any sand. In a large stockpot, bring the water and wine to a boil. Add the quahogs, cover and cook for about 5 minutes, or until the shells open. As they open, remove the clams with tongs and transfer to a large bowl to cool. Discard any clams that do not open. When cool enough to handle, work over a bowl to remove the meat from the clamshells, and place the meat and any juices in a separate bowl.

Add the juices from the cooked clams to the stockpot. Over high heat, bring to a boil, then lower the heat and simmer, uncovered, for 5 minutes to reduce the stock. Place a fine-mesh sieve lined with 2 layers of dampened cheesecloth over a large bowl. Pour the reduced stock through the sieve and set aside.

Clean the stockpot and place it over medium-high heat. Add the butter and when it has melted add the onions and cook until they are tender but not browned. Add the celery, stir and cook for another minute. Pour in the reserved stock from the quahogs, and add the fish stock and herbs. Bring the mixture to a boil. Immediately lower the heat, cover and simmer for about 10 minutes, partially covered.

Add the scallops, shrimp and cubed fish. Bring to a simmer, cover with a tight-fitting lid and cook over medium-low heat for about 3 minutes. While the scallops and fish are cooking, chop the cooked quahog meat and add it to the chowder along with the milk. Season to taste with salt and pepper. Stir and allow the chowder to become thoroughly heated but do not let it boil. Ladle into soup bowls, sprinkle with fresh parsley and serve immediately.

FOR DINNER
Per Serving: Calories 204 • GL 1 • Glycals 1
With a small salad with Caesar dressing: Calories 252 • GL 1 • Glycals 2
❢ Add a glass of white wine: Calories 351 • GL 1 • Glycals 3

FOR LUNCH:
Per Serving: Calories 204 • GL 1 • Glycals 1
With a small salad with Caesar dressing: Calories 252 • GL 1 • Glycals 2
❢ Add a glass of white wine: Calories 351 • GL 1 • Glycals 3

Crab Cakes

Can also be served for lunch (green)

Crab, like all seafood, is low-glycal; it's the cornmeal coating that increases the glycals. As you've learned, the time of day may also affect the rating of the meal. That's why this recipe (with asparagus or with asparagus and wine) is still a green meal at lunch, but a yellow meal at dinner. The crab mixture must be made in advance so the patties can chill for at least an hour before you cook them.

YIELD: 4 SERVINGS

2 lb (910 g) fresh lump crabmeat

¼ cup (40 g) minced onion

¼ cup (30 g) minced celery

¼ cup (35 g) minced red bell pepper

¼ cup (15 g) finely chopped fresh parsley

1 garlic clove, pressed (optional)

3 eggs, beaten

3 tbsp (42 g) melted butter, cooled

1 tsp Worcestershire sauce

2 tbsp (30 ml) fresh lemon juice

Salt and freshly ground black pepper to taste

2 tbsp (18 g) stoneground cornmeal

Vegetable oil, as needed

1 lemon, cut in wedges

Place the crabmeat in a large bowl; pick through it for shell fragments. Add the minced vegetables, parsley and garlic (if using). Toss together. In a separate bowl, whisk together the eggs, butter, Worcestershire sauce, lemon juice, salt and pepper. Add to the crab mixture and combine thoroughly.

Sprinkle half of the cornmeal on a cookie sheet. Form the crab mixture into 4" (10.2-cm) patties (use baking rings, if you have them, set on the cookie sheet to help the patties hold their shape), place on the baking sheet and sprinkle the tops with the remaining cornmeal. Cover with plastic wrap, and refrigerate for at least 1 hour.

When ready to cook, pour vegetable oil into a large, heavy skillet to a depth of ¼" (6 mm). Heat the oil over medium-high heat. When it is hot, but not smoking, add the crab cakes and cook until golden on both sides, turning only once, about 4 minutes per side. If you are cooking the crab cakes in batches, transfer them to a platter in a warm oven. Serve hot with lemon wedges on the side.

Per Serving: Calories 479 • GL 2 • Glycals 10
With asparagus: Calories 518 • GL 3 • Glycals 16
❢ Add a glass of white wine: Calories 617 • GL 3 • Glycals 19

Oyster Spinach Salad

Main course dinner salad

A warm dressing makes this spinach salad special, and the flavors are a perfect complement to fried oysters. Most recipes for fried oysters call for a flour or cornmeal dredge but that one step would change this recipe to high-glycal. Loaded with iron, calcium and Omega-3 fatty acids, this meal-in-one-dish salad is a nutritional powerhouse.

YIELD: 4 SERVINGS

1 red onion, halved and thinly sliced

6 slices bacon, cooked crisp and crumbled

1 cooking apple, peeled and grated

¼ cup (60 ml) cider vinegar

¼ cup (60 ml) dry white wine

¼ tsp dry mustard

Salt and freshly ground black pepper

2 tbsp (28 g) butter

1 lb (455 g) shucked oysters

1 (10 oz [280 g]) bag fresh baby spinach leaves, cleaned

½ cup (60 g) grated Asiago cheese

In a large skillet over medium heat, cook the red onion in 1 tablespoon (15 g) of bacon fat until softened. Add the grated apple and continue cooking for about 1 minute. Add the vinegar, wine, mustard, salt and pepper. Stir well and continue cooking for another 1 minute. Turn off the heat.

In another large skillet, melt the butter over medium-high heat. Add the oysters, without crowding the pan, and cook until golden on both sides. This will take about 2 minutes per side. As they are done, transfer the oysters to an ovenproof plate and place in a warm oven.

To assemble the salad: place the spinach in a large salad bowl with the bacon and cheese. Toss to combine. Pour the warm onion/apple/vinegar dressing over the spinach, and toss.

Divide the dressed spinach among 4 serving plates. Place an equal portion of cooked oysters on each salad. Serve immediately.

Per Serving: Calories 514 • GL 2 • Glycals 9
! Add a glass of white wine: Calories 613 • GL 2 • Glycals 11

Crustless Salmon Quiche

You can make this quiche with fresh poached salmon but canned salmon is excellent and always available on your shelf—and it's an equally good source of omega-3 as well as calcium. For a variation, substitute 2 cups (910 g) of chopped lobster meat or lump crabmeat for the salmon. If you were to pour this filling into a pastry shell (the traditional way to make quiche) this dish becomes high-glycal.

YIELD: 4 SERVINGS

1½ cans wild salmon
(14.75-oz [412-g] each)

3 tbsp (42 g) butter

12 asparagus spears, top
4" (10.2 cm) only of each,
cut into thirds

1 large leek, halved
lengthwise, cleaned and
thinly sliced (white and
pale green part only)

Salt and freshly ground
black pepper, to taste

1 cup (120 g) grated Asiago
cheese, divided

4 eggs

1 cup (235 ml) milk

Preheat oven to 350°F (180°C). Coat a 10-inch (25.4-cm) glass pie dish with cooking spray. Flake the salmon into a mixing bowl.

Melt the butter in a large skillet over medium heat; add the asparagus and leeks to the skillet. Cook over medium-low heat, stirring occasionally, for approximately 7 to 10 minutes or until the asparagus is tender. Season with a little salt and pepper, and add to the bowl of flaked salmon. Add half of the Asiago cheese, and toss the mixture together with a fork to distribute the ingredients evenly. Transfer to the prepared pie dish.

In a bowl, whisk the eggs with the milk. Pour the egg mixture over the salmon mixture. Bake for 15 minutes.

Remove the quiche from the oven carefully. Top the quiche with the remaining ½ cup (60 g) Asiago cheese. Return the quiche to the oven, and continue baking until the quiche is set; approximately 20 minutes more. To test for doneness, insert a knife into the middle of the quiche; it should come out clean. Allow the quiche to stand for 10 minutes before cutting into wedges and serving.

Per Serving: Calories 476 • GL 2 • Glycals 8
With small green salad: Calories 532 • GL 2 • Glycals 11
❢ Add a glass of wine: Calories 631 • GL 2 • Glycals 13
Note: Wine makes this a yellow meal for dinner.

Seared Scallops with Baby Greens

Main course dinner salad

A bed of fresh crisp summer vegetables dressed with a classic vinaigrette and topped with seared-until-golden sea scallops gives a mouthful of sweet, tangy and buttery flavors in every bite.

Many chefs give scallops a quick dusting of flour or cornmeal before dropping them into a hot skillet, but either of those ingredients will increase the glycals in this nutritious dish without improving flavor. So, to keep it low-glycal, we'll skip that step.

The scallops will cook quickly so have all the other parts of this dinner salad prepared first.

YIELD: 4 SERVINGS

DRESSING

2 tbsp (30 ml) fresh lemon juice

½ tsp Dijon mustard

⅓ cup (78 ml) olive oil

1½ tsp (2 g) chopped fresh flat leaf parsley

1½ tsp (2 g) chopped fresh chives

1½ tsp (1 g) chopped fresh basil

Salt and freshly ground black pepper

4 cups (220 g) mixed baby lettuce greens

1 cup (155 g) fresh corn kernels

½ cup (55 g) grated carrots

12 cherry tomatoes, halved

1 tbsp (15 ml) olive oil

1 tbsp (14 g) butter

1 lb (455 g) sea scallops

In a bowl, whisk together all the dressing ingredients. Set aside.

In a large bowl, toss the mixed baby greens with the corn, carrots and cherry tomatoes. Set aside.

In a large, heavy skillet, heat the oil and butter over medium heat. When the butter is sizzling hot, add the scallops and cook until they have a golden crust on both sides, turning only once (use tongs to turn the scallops).

Divide the salad mix among 4 plates. Top each salad with the hot-out-of-the-pan seared scallops. Pour a little dressing over each salad and serve immediately.

Per Serving: Calories 305 • GL 4 • Glycals 11
🍷 Add a glass of white wine: Calories 404 • GL 4 • Glycals 14

Garlic Shrimp

An overnight marinade gives each juicy bite of shrimp a burst of flavor. Shrimp is high in protein, low in calories and available year round—and it's a low-glycal food. Buy wild shrimp, not farmed, whenever possible; the texture and flavor are superior.

After you've let the shrimp marinate, you can finish this dish in 30 minutes, making it great for a main course with a tossed salad of crisp greens and cherry tomatoes, or an hors d'oeuvre for a party.

YIELD: 6 SERVINGS

5 tbsp (70 g) mayonnaise

½ tsp black pepper

5 tbsp (75 ml) fresh lemon juice

4 garlic cloves, minced

2 lb (910 g) uncooked large shrimp, shelled* and deveined

2 tbsp (28 g) melted butter

In a medium bowl, make the marinade by combining the mayonnaise, pepper, lemon juice and garlic; stir until well blended. Place shrimp in a large shallow glass dish. Pour marinade over shrimp, toss until evenly coated with marinade and cover the dish tightly with plastic wrap. Store in refrigerator for a minimum of 4 hours or overnight.

Preheat oven to 400°F (200°C). Place a wire rack in a large shallow baking pan. Remove the shrimp from the marinade and place each one in a single layer on the rack, not touching. Add the melted butter to the reserved marinade and mix together well. With a spoon, dribble a little over each shrimp until all of it is used.

Bake in the preheated oven for 20 minutes, or until the shrimp is opaque. Serve immediately.

***Note:** When you remove the shells from the shrimp, leave them intact at the tail; it adds flavor and makes it easy to pick up the shrimp to eat out of hand if you serve this as an hors d'oeuvre (and at a party, it makes a great one).

Per Serving: Calories 235 • GL 0 • Glycals 0
❢ Add a glass of white wine: Calories 334 • GL 0 • Glycals 0

Tuna Steak Mediterranean

In this simple-to-prepare recipe grilled tuna steaks are topped with a classic combo of Mediterranean flavors—starring tomatoes, olives, oregano and capers—making a delightful dinner on a summer evening. Like all seafood, tuna is high in Omega-3 fatty acids and a low-glycal food. Leftovers? Make them into a low-glycal lunch! For a variation, substitute swordfish for the tuna.

YIELD: 4 SERVINGS

4 (6 oz [168 g]) yellow fin tuna steaks, about ¾" (1.9-cm) thick

Salt and pepper, to taste

1½ cups (270 g) chopped tomato

¼ cup (25 g) chopped scallion

3 tbsp (12 g) chopped fresh parsley

2 tbsp (5 g) chopped fresh basil or oregano leaves

1 tbsp (8.6 g) capers, drained

1 tbsp (15 ml) extra-virgin olive oil

1 tbsp (15 ml) lemon juice

½ tsp minced garlic

12 Kalamata olives, pitted and rough chopped

Heat a large nonstick skillet over medium-high heat. While the skillet gets hot, sprinkle the tuna steaks with salt and pepper. Add the fish to the pan and cook for 4 minutes per side (or longer, depending on your preference for doneness), reducing the heat to medium when you flip the steaks.

While the tuna cooks, combine the chopped tomato, scallion, parsley, basil (or oregano), capers, olive oil, lemon juice, garlic and olives. Mix well.

When the tuna steaks are done, transfer to a plate and top each with a portion of the tomato mixture. Serve immediately.

Per Serving: Calories 454 • GL 1 • Glycals 7
With steamed spinach: Calories 484 • GL 1 • Glycals 7
❢ Add a glass of white wine: Calories 583 • GL 1 • Glycals 8

LOW-GLYCAL DIET SIDE DISHES & SIDE SALADS

Your favorite side dish with dinner may be a simple green salad—good for you—but if you're looking for some fresh ideas for dishes that will go nicely with your new Low-Glycal Diet way of eating, you'll find a terrific selection here. Suggestions on what to pair with these side dishes, as well as how to use the salads at lunch or dinner, are included too, along with, of course, the calories, GL (glycemic load) and glycals for a single serving of each one.

Endive, Fennel and Orange Salad

Crisp, crunchy endive and fennel are complemented well with sweet juicy sections of orange in this simple yet sophisticated salad. Make this during the winter when oranges are at their best and when you'll benefit from the Vitamin C and immune-boosting properties of fennel. These refreshing flavors make this salad a welcome side with a rich roast, and a nice way to round out a low-glycal dinner.

YIELD: 4 SERVINGS

6 tbsp (90 ml) freshly squeezed orange juice

2 tbsp (30 ml) extra-virgin olive oil

Salt and freshly ground black pepper

3 heads endive, trimmed and shredded

1 small fennel bulb, trimmed and sliced paper thin

3 oranges, peel and pith removed and fruit cut into slices, or segments removed whole

In a bowl, whisk together the orange juice, olive oil and salt and pepper.

Place the endive and fennel in a large mixing bowl and toss together. Drizzle the dressing over the greens and toss to coat well.

Divide the salad among 4 plates. Garnish with the orange slices or segments just before serving.

Per Serving: Calories 78 • GL 5 • Glycals 4

Spinach Salad with Bleu Cheese & Red Onions

Dinner side salad

With a bag of fresh baby spinach leaves, there's very little work required to put together this salad. The combination of tender greens and crisp bacon, creamy blue cheese and crunchy sweet-sharp red onion make this nutrient-rich salad a winner with steak or chicken for a low-glycal dinner.

YIELD: 2 SERVINGS

2 cups (110 g) fresh baby spinach leaves, washed

2 slices bacon, cook crisp and crumbled

2 tbsp (16 g) crumbled blue cheese

¼ red onion, thinly sliced

3 tbsp (45 ml) Basic Salad Dressing (recipe on page 183)

Place the spinach in a salad bowl and add the bacon, blue cheese and red onion. Toss well, add the salad dressing and toss again. Serve immediately.

Per Serving: Calories 359 • GL 1 • Glycals 3

Caesar Salad

Crisp Romaine lettuce, a mouth-puckering dressing, a dusting of buttery Parmesan, and a chewy anchovy or two makes a delightful salad-lunch on its own, or in a smaller portion as a side salad at dinner. You can turn it into a main course dinner salad by topping it with grilled or boiled shrimp, sliced roasted chicken breast or sliced grilled flank steak—and it's still a green meal. Another plus: the dressing is made in a blender!

Traditional Caesar salad contains croutons, which changes the recipe from low-glycal to high-glycal, so they are not included here. You won't miss them!

YIELD: 2 SERVINGS

---

1 head Romaine lettuce, cleaned and trimmed

1 egg

2 tbsp (30 ml) fresh lemon juice

10 anchovy filets

1 garlic clove

3 tbsp (45 ml) olive oil

¼ tsp Worcestershire sauce

Salt and freshly ground black pepper, to taste

⅓ cup (66 g) grated Parmesan cheese

Remove and discard any tough outer leaves from the Romaine lettuce; cut off the base; remove and discard the core of small white leaves (these are bitter). Plunge the remaining lettuce leaves into a salad spinner filled with cold water, let sit for 2 minutes, drain and spin dry. Lay the leaves on paper towels or a clean kitchen towel; roll the toweling loosely around the lettuce and store in the refrigerator while you make the dressing.

In a small bowl, whisk the egg and lemon juice together; let sit for 5 minutes.

Place 4 anchovy filets in a blender with the garlic, olive oil, Worcestershire sauce and the egg/lemon mixture. Blend until smooth. Season to taste with salt and pepper.

Tear the lettuce into rough pieces and place in a salad bowl. Pour the dressing over the top and toss well. Add the cheese, and toss again. Divide the salad into two portions, top each with three anchovy filets and serve.

Per Serving: Calories 242 • GL 1 • Glycals 3

FOR A SIDE SALAD AT DINNER:
Yield: 4 Servings
Per Serving: Calories 125 • GL 1 • Glycals 1

Guacamole

Lunch or dinner side dish

If you've ever been on a weight-loss diet that didn't allow avocados, good news—they are a low-glycal food! As creamy as their texture is, avocados are a good source of fiber and a powerhouse of healthy fats and vitamins. Guacamole—a mashed avocado dish brightened with notes of lime, garlic and cilantro—is a key ingredient in all kinds of wraps, as you'll see in some of the recipes in this book. It is also a tasty side dish full of good-for-you fats that help you feel full. Make guacamole right before you plan on serving it; it loses a lot once refrigerated.

YIELD: 8 SERVINGS

4 large ripe avocados, peeled and pitted

3 limes, juice only

2 medium-size tomatoes, chopped

1 small onion, minced

2 garlic cloves, minced

½ serrano or jalapeño chili pepper, seeded and minced

3 tbsp (3 g) chopped fresh cilantro

Salt and freshly ground black pepper to taste

In a mixing bowl, mash the avocados with a fork. Mix in the remaining ingredients, and serve.

Per Serving: Calories 50 • GL 0 • Glycals 0

Brussels Sprouts with Bacon

Dinner side dish

Brussels sprouts are a terrific low-glycal choice for a side dish during the fall and winter, when they are in season and at their most flavorful. A member of the cabbage family, this highly flavorful vegetable is an excellent source of vitamins (particularly vitamin C), protein, dietary fiber and a compound believed to have anti-cancer properties. No wonder it's considered a "power food!" Complemented with the rich taste of bacon, this side dish goes very well with roasted chicken or a grilled steak, and can also be used as a topping for a winter dinner salad.

YIELD: 4 SERVINGS

---

1 lb (455 g) fresh Brussels sprouts, rinsed, stems trimmed

Place the Brussels sprouts in a large pot of cold water and set over high heat.

¼ lb (115 g) bacon, chopped (apple wood smoked bacon is a great choice for this recipe)

As soon as the water reaches a boil, set a timer for 2 minutes. Drain and rinse them under cold water to stop the cooking process. Set aside in a colander.

Salt and freshly ground black pepper

Place the bacon in a large skillet set over medium-high heat. Sauté the bacon until it has started to become brown and crisp. Remove pan from heat and spoon off and discard half of the rendered bacon fat. Return the skillet to the heat and add the Brussels sprouts. Toss gently and season with a little salt and freshly ground black pepper. Continue cooking until the Brussels sprouts are piping hot and tender; serve immediately.

Per Serving: Calories 171 • GL 0.5 • Glycals 3.5

Roasted Brussels Sprouts

Dinner side dish

If you grew up thinking you didn't like Brussels sprouts, it may be because you only had them boiled to death. Roasted, however, this little green globe takes on a sweet nutty flavor that complements any rich, fatty meat. Topped with a high-quality balsamic vinegar, you have a low-glycal dish that's high in antioxidants!

YIELD: 4 SERVINGS

1 lb (455 g) fresh Brussels sprouts, rinsed, stems trimmed and halved (cut through stem end)

2 tbsp (30 ml) olive oil

Salt and pepper to taste

2 tbsp (30 ml) balsamic vinegar

Preheat oven to 375°F (190°C). Prepare the Brussels sprouts right before cooking so that there is still some water on them from being rinsed.

Set an oven-proof skillet over medium heat, add the oil and when it is hot, but not smoking, add the Brussels sprouts. Add a little salt and pepper, toss quickly so the sprouts are all coated with a bit of the oil, cover the skillet with a tight-fitting lid and lower the heat to low. Set a timer for 2 minutes.

Remove the lid and raise the heat to medium. Cook for another minute. Transfer the skillet to the preheated oven and cook, uncovered, for 10 minutes. Check the sprouts for tenderness and continue cooking for another 3 to 5 minutes if they are too firm.

When cooked to desired tenderness, remove from the oven and sprinkle with the balsamic vinegar. Toss and serve immediately.

Per Serving: Calories 171 • GL: 0.5 • Glycals 3.5

Savory Sautéed Savoy Cabbage

Savoy cabbage is the one with the crinkly surface on its leaves. Savoy is tender and sweet, much more so than the standard smooth-leaved cabbage, as a matter of fact. It can even be enjoyed raw, as a "wrap" instead of bread for a sandwich. Here, it's complimented with garlic and scallions. A whole head of cabbage keeps well in the fridge, and as a member of the cruciferous family of vegetables, it is considered a superfood. It's good with pork or lamb, and it's low-glycal.

YIELD: 4 SERVINGS

3 tbsp (45 ml) olive oil

6 scallions, chopped

2 garlic cloves, chopped

1 head Savoy cabbage, cored and thinly sliced

Salt and freshly ground black pepper

¼ cup (60 ml) water

Heat the oil in a 12-inch (30.5-cm) skillet over medium heat until it is hot, but not smoking. Add the white part of the scallions and the garlic to the oil, stirring occasionally, and cook until the garlic is a pale gold, about 2 minutes. Add the cabbage, season with salt and pepper and raise the heat to medium-high. Use tongs to turn the cabbage, and sauté for 1 minute. Add the water, cover with a tight-fitting lid and cook until the cabbage wilts, about 3 minutes.

Add the green part of the scallions and cook, uncovered, until most of the water has evaporated and the cabbage is tender, about 2 minutes, tossing occasionally with tongs. Season to taste with additional salt and pepper and serve.

Per Serving: Calories 123 • GL 1 • Glycals 1

Red Cabbage with Caraway Seeds

Dinner side dish

Cabbage makes a great side dish with pork but it's also very good with turkey. Here, the cabbage is cooked until tender-crisp and enhanced with the anise-like flavor and chewy texture of caraway. This low-glycal recipe goes together quickly, making it a great choice for a weeknight dinner. And, it's so simple, after you've made it once you'll pull it off without even referring to the recipe. Need another reason to try it? Red cabbage is an excellent source of vitamins K and C, and high in fiber.

YIELD: 4 SERVINGS

---

4 cups (220 g) shredded red cabbage

2 tbsp (30 ml) fresh lemon juice, divided

3 tbsp (45 ml) olive oil

5 tbsp (75 ml) chicken broth or vegetable broth

1 shallot, minced

1 tsp caraway seeds—or more, to taste

Salt and freshly ground black pepper, to taste

Place the cabbage in a large bowl, sprinkle with 1 tablespoon (30 ml) of the lemon juice, toss and set aside.

Heat the oil in a large skillet set over medium heat. When it is hot and shimmering, but not smoking, add the cabbage and cover with a tight-fitting lid. Cook, covered, for 5 minutes.

Transfer the cooked cabbage to a large bowl. While still hot, toss the cabbage with the remaining ingredients. Let it sit for 5 minutes. Toss again, and serve.

Per Serving: Calories 86 • GL 1 • Glycals 1

Roasted Cauliflower with Capers

Dinner side dish

The golden color of the cauliflower florets is only the first attractive thing about this recipe. It's mild yet earthy flavor is enhanced with fresh lemon juice and the tangy bite of capers. High in vitamin C and sulforaphane (a cancer-fighting compound), cauliflower goes especially well with lamb. Try this with a grilled lamb shoulder chop or with a swordfish steak. Add a small green salad and you've got a delicious low-glycal dinner.

YIELD: 4 SERVINGS

2 tbsp (30 ml) olive oil

1 head cauliflower, base trimmed, broken into florets

Salt and freshly ground black pepper

1 lemon, juiced

2 tbsp (17 g) capers

Preheat oven to 350°F (180°C). Heat the oil in a heavy oven-proof skillet over medium-high heat and when it is hot, but not smoking, add the cauliflower. Toss quickly so that all pieces are coated with oil, and season with a little salt and pepper. Continue cooking just until the florets have golden edges, then transfer to the hot oven and roast for 15 to 20 minutes or until the cauliflower is the desired tenderness.

Remove from the oven and pour the juice of a freshly squeezed lemon over the cauliflower. Toss. Add the capers and toss again. Serve hot.

Per Serving: Calories 78 • GL 1 • Glycals 1

Cauliflower Casserole

Dinner side dish

The gooey, cheesy, golden topping of this casserole is the perfect lid for the tender cauliflower in tomato sauce that lies under it. An excellent source of vitamin C, cauliflower is classified as one of the top 10 "healthiest foods." You can assemble this dish in advance, if you like; store it in the fridge and bake it when you're ready. Let the casserole sit on the counter while you preheat the oven so it does not go in cold.

YIELD: 4 SERVINGS

1 large cauliflower, base trimmed and head broken into florets

Salt and freshly ground black pepper

1 cup (245 g) tomato sauce

½ cup (60 g) grated Gruyère or Swiss cheese

2 tbsp (28 g) butter, cut into small pieces

Preheat oven to 350°F (180°C). Bring a large pot of lightly salted water to a boil. Add the cauliflower pieces to the boiling water; as soon as the water returns to a boil, set a timer for 2 minutes. Pour into a colander and let the cauliflower drain.

Place the cauliflower in a wide shallow casserole dish and season with salt and pepper. Pour the tomato sauce over it, sprinkle the cheese evenly over the top and then dot with the butter. Cover with foil and bake for 20 minutes. Remove the foil and continue baking for another 5 to 7 minutes or until the cheese is bubbly and golden brown.

Per Serving: Calories 138 • GL 2 • Glycals 3

Garlic Roasted Green Beans

Dinner side dish

Green beans are a versatile low-glycal food, rich in B vitamins and carotenoids, that can be enjoyed hot, cold or at room temperature in a variety of ways. This simple yet flavorful recipe is quick to prepare and the garlic and Parmesan makes it one that goes well with chicken, pork, beef, lamb or seafood. Pair this side dish with any single serving of grilled or roasted meat, a small salad lightly dressed, and you will have a satisfying low-glycal dinner.

Any leftovers make a great mid-afternoon snack, too.

YIELD: 4 SERVINGS

1½ lb (680 g) green beans, cleaned and trimmed

2 cloves garlic, peeled and thinly sliced

2 tbsp (30 ml) extra-virgin olive oil

Salt and pepper

2 tbsp (10 g) Parmesan cheese

Preheat oven to 425°F (220°C). Place the green beans in a shallow, rimmed baking dish. Add the garlic, olive oil and season with a pinch of salt and a few grinds of pepper. Toss together.

Bake for approximately 15 minutes, or until the green beans are lightly caramelized but still slightly crisp.

Remove from the oven, sprinkle with the Parmesan cheese and serve.

Per Serving: Calories 121 • GL 1 • Glycals 1

Green Bean Salad with Fontina Cheese

Dinner side dish

Serve this green bean salad slightly chilled so that the tender-crisp texture of the beans can be enjoyed as a crunchy mouthful. The mild yet nutty flavor of the Fontina cheese adds a slightly sweet note and soft texture to a salad that is pulled together with a classic vinaigrette. It makes a great low-glycal side dish for summer meals.

YIELD: 4 SERVINGS

1 lb (455 g) green beans, cleaned and trimmed

½ lb (225 g) Fontina cheese, grated

1 garlic clove, minced

½ tsp Dijon mustard

¼ cup (60 ml) lemon juice

¼ cup (60 ml) olive oil

Salt and freshly ground black pepper, to taste

Bring a large pot of lightly salted water to a boil. Add the beans and set a timer for 2 minutes. Immediately pour the beans into a colander set under cold running water to stop the cooking process. Drain; let sit while you grate the cheese.

Transfer the beans to a large bowl and add the cheese. Toss gently.

In a separate small bowl, whisk together the garlic and mustard. Add the lemon juice and whisk well. Slowly add the oil, whisking constantly. Pour the dressing over the beans and cheese. Toss gently. Season to taste with salt and pepper. Cover and refrigerate until ready to serve.

Per Serving: Calories 316 • GL 1 • Glycals 3

Green Bean Salad with Walnuts

Lunch or dinner side dish

The directions for cooking the green beans for this salad yield a crisp bean. If you like yours a little more tender, leave in the boiling water for up to 2 minutes but no longer. Served chilled or at room temperature, the crisp beans are perfectly complemented by the rich flavors of buttery toasted walnuts and Gorgonzola cheese. This dish is excellent with any meat or seafood.

YIELD: 4 SERVINGS

1 lb (455 g) fresh green beans, cleaned, trimmed, and cut into 1" (25-cm) pieces

½ cup (60 g) walnuts, lightly toasted

½ cup (60 g) Gorgonzola cheese, crumbled

3 scallions, thinly sliced, white and pale green only

3 tbsp (45 ml) Basic Salad Dressing (recipe on page 183)

Bring a large pot of lightly salted water to a boil. Add the green beans, cover and as soon as the water returns to a boil drain the beans into a colander. Set aside to cool. At this point, you could refrigerate the beans in a covered dish until you are ready to finish the salad.

When the beans have cooled, place them in a salad bowl with the walnuts, cheese and scallions. Toss together gently. Pour the dressing over the salad and toss again.

Serve immediately.

Per Serving: Calories 396 • GL 1 • Glycals 4

Herbed Green Beans

Dinner side dish

Green beans go well with a variety of low-glycal main courses so it's handy to have a few ways to prepare them. Here, the sweet, mellow tastes of balsamic vinegar and aromatic rosemary bring out a side of green beans you didn't know existed. This simple recipe goes together quickly and can be served hot or at room temperature.

YIELD: 4 SERVINGS

1 lb (455 g) green beans, trimmed but not cut

1 tbsp (15 ml) balsamic vinegar

2 tsp (10 ml) olive oil

½ tsp dried rosemary leaves, finely crushed

½ tsp dried thyme leaves

¼ tsp salt

Pinch freshly ground black pepper

Place the green beans in a medium saucepan and add enough water to cover them; place over high heat. When the water reaches a boil, reduce heat to low, and simmer for 3 to 4 minutes or until the beans are tender but still crisp. Drain. Return the beans to the saucepan.

Add the vinegar, oil, herbs, salt and pepper to the beans. Toss and cook over medium heat for 1 to 2 minutes or until heated through.

Per Serving: Calories 56 • GL 1 • Glycals 0

Parmesan Potatoes

Breakfast, brunch or dinner

Sometimes, you just want potatoes! When you are in Step 2 or Step 3 of the diet, you can have a red dish, so work this one into your meal plan if you know you'll be craving potatoes. With their crisp golden edges, you'll swear these potatoes were fried in a skillet but the beauty part is this side dish cooks in the oven for an hour.

YIELD: 8 SERVINGS

6 medium-size Russet potatoes

½ cup (50 g) grated Parmesan cheese

¼ cup (32 g) flour

1 tsp salt

1 tsp pepper

4 tbsp (55 g) butter

Preheat oven to 350°F (180°C). Peel the potatoes, and cut each into 8 pieces. Combine the cheese, flour, salt and pepper in a paper bag. In batches, place the potatoes in the bag, hold the top shut and shake.

Put the butter into a 9 x 13-inch (23 cm x 33-cm) pan. Place the pan in the preheated oven until the butter melts. Remove the pan and add the coated potatoes. Bake, uncovered, for 30 minutes.

Use a metal spatula to turn the potatoes over, being careful not to dislodge the crust that will have developed on the bottom. Bake for an additional 20 to 30 minutes, or until the potatoes are golden brown on all sides. Serve hot.

Per Serving: Calories 178 • GL 20 • Glycals 32

Vegetable Gratin

Dinner side dish

This low-glycal recipe is a tasty way to use summer produce. And, because it can be served at room temperature, it's handy for a buffet. The layers of zucchini, tomato and eggplant almost melt into each other, creating a juicy, savory side dish that goes well with any meat or fish.

YIELD: 6 SERVINGS

1 medium-size zucchini, unpeeled, sliced ¼" (6-mm) thick

4 large tomatoes, sliced ¼" (6-mm) thick

1 eggplant, unpeeled, sliced ¼" (6-mm) thick

½ cup (60 ml) of extra-virgin olive oil

1 garlic clove, very thinly sliced

Salt and freshly ground black pepper

3 tbsp (7.5 g) fresh chopped basil

Preheat oven to 350°F (180°C). Lightly oil a 9- or 10-inch (23- or 25.4-cm) diameter shallow baking dish. Starting at the outside edge, arrange the vegetables in concentric circles to the center of the dish, alternating pieces of zucchini, tomato and eggplant.

When all the vegetables have been used, pour the olive oil over the vegetables evenly; distribute the garlic evenly over all and season with salt and pepper. Cover the dish with foil and place in the hot oven.

Bake, covered, for 15 minutes. Remove the foil and bake for an additional 10 minutes or until the vegetables are tender and juicy. Remove from the oven and sprinkle with the fresh basil. Serve hot, or at room temperature.

Per Serving: Calories 113 • GL 1 • Glycals 1

Basic Salad Dressing

Once you make this dressing and any of the suggested variations, you'll never buy bottled dressing again. Why is that a good thing? Most bottled dressings contain sugar or high-fructose corn syrup, both of which are high-glycal. Plus, you can use top-quality olive oil when you make your own dressing, a flavorful vinegar and the fresh or dried herbs of your choice.

YIELD: 1 CUP (A SINGLE SERVING IS A TABLESPOON [15 ML])

⅓ cup (78 ml) apple cider vinegar

⅔ cup (157 ml) extra-virgin olive oil

1 tsp Dijon mustard

1 garlic clove or 1 small shallot

½ tsp salt

A few grinds of black pepper

Combine all ingredients in blender. Taste and season as needed. You can add 1 tablespoon (15 ml) of fresh lemon juice if the dressing is not zippy enough. Or add more oil if it is too tangy.

Store in the fridge in a glass jar, tightly covered (do not store in plastic!) but bring to room temperature and shake well before using.

Per Serving: Calories: 158 • GL 0 • Glycals 0

VARIATIONS

Tarragon: add to the blender 1 tablespoon (4.8 g) dried tarragon, crushed

Cheese: add to the blender ⅓ cup (40 g) Gorgonzola cheese, or blue cheese, or grated Parmesan

Mediterranean: add to the blender 3 anchovies

Quick Caesar: add to the blender 3 anchovies, 1 teaspoon Worchestershire sauce and ½ cup (50 g) grated Parmesan

LOW-GLYCAL DIET SNACK RECIPES

You don't need a recipe for most of the low-glycal snacks you've seen suggested in the meal plans for Step 1, 2 and 3 of the low-glycal diet. But you probably noticed that some of the snacks made reference to a recipe. The handful of recipes here are simple to prepare and offer a distinct departure from a snack of a fresh apple or handful of nuts. I hope you'll try them and find some that you love.

By the way, the Hummus, Savory Cheese Spread and Marseille-Style Sardine Dip all make excellent hors d'oeuvres. So, the next time you're having a party, think about putting one of those out with your other offerings.

If you are in the habit of reaching for a bag of chips or crackers when there is a dip or spread to snack on, you will want to change that habit as you become a glycal-conscious eater. The solution: endive, or Belgian endive as it is sometimes called, is a small tight head of narrow canoe-shaped, smooth, crisp leaves. (You'll find it in the lettuce display at your market.) Once the base is trimmed, each leaf is about 5 inches (12.7-cm) long. The base end of each leaf forms a scoop that is crisp enough to act as a "dipper," making it a perfect replacement for chips and crackers. Its delicate taste does not interfere with the favor of whatever you're spreading on it (or dipping it into), either. And, it's low-glycal!

TO SNACK OR NOT TO SNACK? THAT IS THE QUESTION.

The answer: Yes, by all means, have a snack! Snacks are an important part of the Low-Glycal Diet, which is why they are included in each of the meal plans. Your snacks should be low-glycal (unless you are in Step 2 or Step 3 and you have planned a medium- or high-glycal snack as part of a day's menu), and they should be separated from your meals by 2 hours. But, that doesn't mean you can only have two snacks a day. If, for example, you eat lunch at noon and are finished 30 minutes later, you could have a snack at 2:30 p.m., another snack at 4:30 p.m. and dinner at 6:30 p.m. If the snacks are low-glycal, you won't be storing fat and you won't be famished when you finally do sit down for dinner. This is particularly important during the phase when you are still losing weight; don't let unnecessary hunger sabotage all your good work. Go ahead, have some Cheese Sticks!

Cheese Sticks

If you like cheese, having it for a mid-morning or mid-afternoon snack while you're on a weight-loss diet is a treat, and very satisfying—not to mention a great source of calcium. Why not cut up a pound (455 g) of cheese at a time and have a few days' worth of cheese sticks ready to go?

YIELD: 4 SERVINGS

8½ oz (240 g) of any hard or firm cheese (Swiss, cheddar, Gouda, Muenster, mozzarella, etc.)

Using a sharp, heavy knife, divide the cheese into 4 equal portions. Cut each portion into French fry-like sticks. Wrap each single portion well in plastic wrap and store in fridge until ready to eat.

Per Serving: Calories: 250* • GL 0 • Glycals 0
*A serving of cheddar cheese has 250 calories; Swiss has 228, Gouda has 226, Muenster has 221, and mozzarella has 154. All have zero GL and zero glycals.

Savory Cheese Spread

Wondering what to do with the miscellaneous small hunks of cheese in your fridge? Get out the food processor and make this savory spread because cheese is a low-glycal food and makes a filling snack, plus it's a great source of calcium. Use this recipe as a guide; once you've made this spread, you'll see how easy it is to improvise the cheeses and measurements. The spread can be packed into custard dishes, covered well in plastic wrap and frozen. Defrost overnight in the fridge.

YIELD: 4 SERVINGS

¼ cup (25 g) Swiss cheese, grated

¼ cup (30 g) cheddar cheese, grated

¼ cup (50 g) goat cheese, crumbled

¼ cup (30 g) bleu cheese or Gorgonzola cheese, crumbled

2 tbsp (10 g) Parmesan cheese, grated

2–4 tbsp (30–60 g) cream cheese

2 tbsp (30 ml) white wine

Dash of Worcestershire sauce

1 garlic clove, finely minced, or 1 small shallot, finely minced (1 tbsp [10 g])

1 tbsp (14 g) softened butter

Grate or chop up the hard cheeses and place them along with all the other ingredients in the bowl of a food processor fitted with the metal blade. Pulse, until you have a smooth spread. Transfer to a bowl, cover well with plastic wrap, and refrigerate for at least 4 hours to allow the spread to become firm. Serve with endive or other crisp raw vegetables.

Note: A dollop of this spread on top of a sizzling hot steak or lamb chop is delicious.

Per Serving: Calories 122 • GL 0 • Glycals 0

Hummus

Hummus—a smooth puree of cooked chickpeas—is available in the fresh-prepared foods section of most supermarkets, but it's easy to make your own and, when you do, you can make it as garlicky or lemony or spicy as you like. Hummus is typically spread on pita bread but on the low-glycal diet you will be avoiding bread because it's a high-glycal food. Instead, enjoy this high-fiber, high-protein dip on endive leaves (the perfect crisp scoop) or celery stems. (You will need a food processor or powerful blender to make this dish.)

YIELD: 9 SERVINGS

4 garlic cloves

2 cups (480 g) canned chickpeas, drained and rinsed

1½ tsp (7.5 g) kosher salt

⅓ cup (80 g) tahini (sesame paste)

4 tbsp (60 ml) fresh lemon juice

3 tbsp (45 ml) olive oil

1 tsp cumin

2 tbsp (8 g) chopped fresh flat leaf parsley

Turn on the food processor fitted with the steel blade and drop the garlic down the feed tube; process until it's minced. Add all the other ingredients except the parsley and pulse until the mixture is smooth. Transfer to a bowl and stir in the parsley. Taste for seasoning, cover and store in the fridge for up to one week. Serve at room temperature.

Per Serving: Calories 70 • GL 3 • Glycals 2

Marseille-Style Sardine Spread

Sardines are a tasty little saltwater fish, high in protein and Omega-3 fatty acids (excellent for brain and heart health), and a good source of calcium, too. They are easy to keep on hand, and because they are sold in small sealed tins that stack neatly, I like to buy a half-dozen at a time. Sardines come packed in a variety of ways: in olive oil, tomato sauce, mustard sauce or water, all of which still give you a low-glycal food.

This dip can be made up to 2 days in advance and stored in the fridge in a tightly sealed glass container. It makes a great low-glycal mid-morning or afternoon snack, and there's plenty here for more than one serving. The seafood flavor—think: tuna with an attitude—is pleasing but not overly assertive.

YIELD: 6 SERVINGS

2 cans of sardines (3.75-oz [106-g] each), packed in tomato sauce

4 tbsp (55 g) softened butter

3 tbsp (45 ml) fresh lemon juice

Salt and freshly ground black pepper to taste

1 head endive, rinsed and separated

Place the sardines and butter in the bowl of a food processor and pulse until well combined (you can also do this by hand in a mixing bowl with a fork). Gradually add the lemon juice, stopping when the dip reaches a soft but not runny consistency. Season to taste with salt and pepper. Transfer to a dish, cover and chill. The mixture will firm once chilled.

Serve with endive, using the white end of the leaf as a spoon to hold the spread.

Per Serving: Calories 112 • GL 2.5 • Glycals 2.5

Tzatziki Dip

This tasty combination of tart creamy yogurt and cool crisp cucumber makes for a delightfully refreshing zero-glycal summertime snack with fresh vegetables, or a flavorful dressing over a bed of salad greens. The fresh dill and mint are a must (do not use dried).

YIELD: 6 SERVINGS

Half of one large English cucumber, coarsely chopped (approx. 1¼ cups [165 g])

1 tsp salt

1 garlic clove, minced

2 tbsp (30 ml) fresh lemon juice

1 tsp fresh dill

1 tsp fresh mint

Freshly ground black pepper, to taste

1½ cups (345 g) Greek yogurt, plain

Place the cucumber in a colander set over a bowl, sprinkle with salt and cover with a small plate weighted with a heavy coffee mug. Let sit for 30 minutes; this allows the cucumber to release some liquid, which will keep the dip from becoming runny. Toss the drained cucumber quickly in a paper towel to further dry it.

Place the cucumber in a food processor with the garlic, lemon juice, dill, mint and a few grinds of black pepper. Pulse quickly until you have a consistent blend that retains distinct pieces of cucumber. Transfer to a bowl and stir in the yogurt. Season to taste with salt and more pepper. Cover and refrigerate for at least 2 hours before serving to allow the flavors to develop. Serve with carrot or celery sticks, or endive. (Keeps well for a few days in the fridge. Drain off any excess liquid that accumulates and stir well before serving.)

Per Serving: Calories 43 • GL 1 • Glycals 0

CHAPTER 8

THERE'S AN APP FOR THAT—CHECKING YOUR MEALS WITH THE REVOLUTIONARY LOW-GLYCAL DIET APP

As you have seen in the previous chapters, there is more to losing fat than just counting calories. Calories count, no doubt about it, but there are times when you can eat all the calories you want and not store fat. There are also times when you'll store more than half the calories you eat as fat. If you want to lose *fat*, and not muscle, you need to consider all the factors important in fat storage and metabolism. To review, these are:

1. The total calories in your meals

2. The total glycemic *load* (not glycemic *index*) of your meals

3. The portion size of each meal

4. The timing between your meals

5. The time of day you eat your meals

6. How much sleep you get each night

Most diets only count calories; a few consider glycemic *index*; but hardly any take into account glycemic *load*, which is critical for fat loss. Only **The Low Glycal Diet**™ incorporates how calories and glycemic *load* interact, how the portion size of your meal affects fat storage, and how the timing of the meals and the amount of sleep you get each night come into play. This is why most diets only partially work; they fail to address the full picture. They are the diets of the past. It's easy to count calories or keep track of the glycemic index of the foods you eat, but it's not so easy to translate the glycemic index of the foods you eat into the glycemic load of your meals and—without some help—it's impossible to calculate how calories and glycemic load interact. Luckily, that help is probably in your pocket or purse right now.

HELP IS A FINGER-TAP AWAY

Today, almost everyone has a smartphone. Smartphones can do wonderful things, but most people barely scratch the surface of their potential. In addition to being a phone and a high-definition video recorder, there are mobile apps that keep you connected through social networks, allow you to take free online courses and listen to lectures, access satellite photographs giving you a birds-eye view of almost any location on earth—and the list goes on.

There are also diet apps—lots of them. A quick search for "diet" at the Apple App Store yields more than 5,000 diet apps. Unfortunately, most diet app developers are not physicians or scientists, so their apps are just a rehashing of the diets of the past. Some of the most popular diet apps only add up the calories you eat and the calories you burn, or give you a host of features that are unimportant when it comes to figuring out how to lose fat. With those apps, you can spend hours a day inputting variables that are completely irrelevant.

That's why, in 2012, I developed The Low Glycal Diet™ Calculator and Tracker. And, now that I've written this book, The Low Glycal Diet™ Calculator and Tracker app serves as the perfect companion for it. Now, you can supplement the meal plans and recipes in the book with your own recipes, and check them easily with the app. You can also put your own spin on the recipes in the book and, with the use of the app, make sure they remain "green." I've taken all of the latest research on fat loss and made it easily accessible and usable with the app. You don't have to count calories, glycemic load or even worry about when you eat your meal; the app does it all for you.

If you haven't downloaded the app yet, I want you to take a moment and do it now. It's free! Just go to the Apple App Store or Google Play (depending on the type of smart phone you have), and search for "Low Glycal Diet." Once the home screen for the app appears (it's pictured below), press "Get" at the Apple App Store or "Install" at Google Play. It only takes a minute to download to your phone and, as I mentioned, it's free. More than 100,000 people around the world have downloaded it to date. The app has helped my patients, as well as tens of thousands of people across the globe, achieve effortless fat loss.

To make it fun and interesting, I've made the app like a game. You assemble meals and check them to see if they're "green," "yellow" or "red." If the meal is "yellow" or "red," the app will highlight the worst food in the meal so you can remove it and substitute a different food, or decrease the serving size. You can continue to switch foods in and out of a meal until you get a "green." You don't even need to understand the science; if you stay "in the green," you'll lose fat. But, if you understand the science—which you learned in the first two chapters of this book—you'll soon be able to spot bad combinations of foods without even using the app, making it more likely that you'll follow the diet.

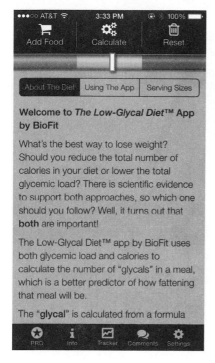

The app is user-friendly and highly visual. There are more than 1,000 easy-to-find foods that are color-coded as green (low-glycal), yellow (medium-glycal) or red (high-glycal) when eaten *alone*. To assemble a meal, just touch the **Add Food** icon. A menu will appear with buttons for 10 different food categories. There are also buttons for favorite foods and favorite meals, which you can create as you use the app. Touching a food category will give you a drop down menu with all the foods in that category. Touching the food will then add it to your meal. You can also search for a food by touching the **Search for a Food** button near the top of the screen. The serving size of each food can be adjusted by touching the "+"or "–" icon below the food.

When you've added all the foods you're thinking about eating to the meal, touch the **Calculate** icon and it will compute the total number of calories, the total glycemic load and the total number of glycals in that meal, and give you a green, yellow or red result on the colored bar at the top. If you get a yellow or red result, the app will highlight the food with the highest number of glycals. You can remove that food easily from the meal by touching the **Remove This Food** icon, and add a different food, or you can adjust the serving size. Touching the **Calculate** icon again will recalculate the meal. Touching the **Reset** icon will allow you to start over again.

For example, if you wanted to have bacon and eggs for breakfast, you'd touch the Add Food button to bring up the categories of food.

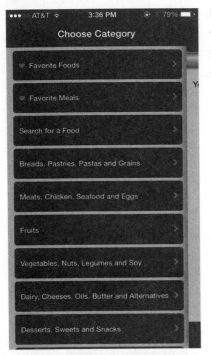

If you go down to the category of Meats, Chicken, Seafood and Eggs and touch that button, a drop down menu with all the choices will appear.

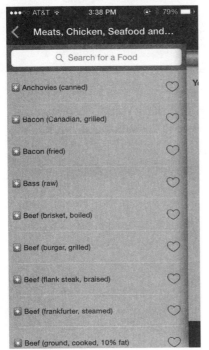

You can add bacon to the meal by touching that entry in the food list.

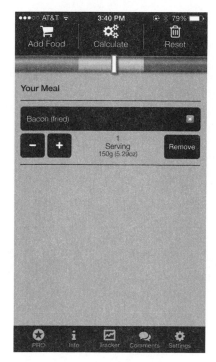

You can adjust the serving size by touching the "-" or "+" buttons below the food. For purposes of the app, the serving sizes of the different foods are listed below.

Breads, Pastries, Pastas and Grains:

- One slice of bread (need 2 servings for a sandwich)
- One bagel, baguette or muffin
- One bowl of cereal
- One cup of pasta, rice or quinoa
- One handful of seeds

Meat, Chicken, Seafood and Eggs:

- One piece of meat, poultry or fish about the size of a deck of cards
- One large egg
- Two slices of cheese or ½ cup (115 g) of cottage cheese

Fruits

- One medium-sized apple, peach, pear or banana
- One slice of watermelon or pineapple: ½ of a larger fruit like cantaloupe
- One handful of berries, grapes, raisins or other dried fruit

Vegetables, Nuts, Legumes and Soy

- One cup (100 g) of cooked vegetables or beans
- One handful of nuts (¼ cup [36 g])
- One medium-sized potato or sweet potato

Dairy, Cheeses, Oils and Butter

- A twelve ounce (355-ml) glass of milk
- One tablespoon (30 g) of cream, butter, margarine, mayonnaise or oil
- One cup of ice cream (140 g) or yogurt (230 g)

Desserts, Sweets and Snacks

- One medium piece of cake or pie
- One candy bar, cookie or doughnut
- One small bag of chips, crackers or pretzels

Drinks

- Eight ounces (235 ml) of juice
- Twelve ounces (355 ml) of milk, soda or beer
- Sixteen ounces (475 ml) of a smoothie or protein drink
- One glass of wine; one shot of hard liquor

Condiments, Spices, Sugar and Sweeteners

- One tablespoon (15 g) of sugar, artificial sweetener
- One tablespoon (15 g) of ketchup, mustard or soy sauce
- Two tablespoons (30 g) of peanut butter, guacamole, honey, jam or maple syrup
- One teaspoon of herbs or spice

Sauces, Salad Dressings and Soups

- Two tablespoons of salad dressing (30 ml)
- One cup (235 ml) of soup
- ½ cup (125 g) of sauce

Prepared and Fast Foods

- One medium slice of pizza
- One cup of macaroni and cheese
- Two pieces of sushi
- Actual serving sizes of fast foods

If you want less than a full serving, you can change the serving size to one-half, one-quarter or one-eighth of a serving using the "+" or "-" button on the app. In this case, we'll adjust the serving size of bacon to ½ of a serving, or about 2.65 ounces (75 g).

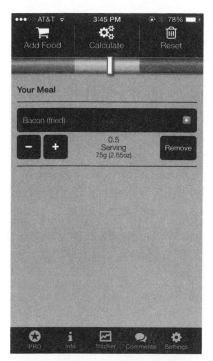

If you want to add a food in the same category, like eggs, just swipe to the right to get the food list again and scroll down to eggs.

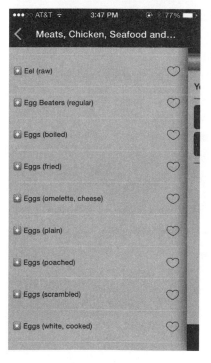

Choose the type of egg and touch it to add it to the meal. You can adjust the number of eggs you're having by touching the "-" or "+" buttons again. In our example, we'll add three scrambled eggs.

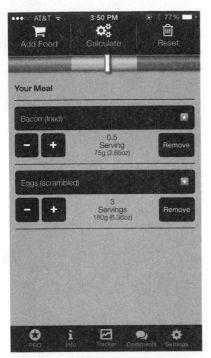

If that's all you're having, touch the calculate button at the top to calculate the meal.

The app will give you a green, yellow or red rating, based on how many calories you'll store as fat.

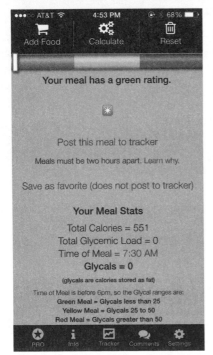

You can see that this meal is "green." It has 551 calories, but the glycemic load is zero. This means the meal doesn't spike your blood sugar, so there's no insulin surge and none of the calories will be stored as fat. From our rotary analogy, we know that if the calories cannot be stored as fat (the entrance gate to the parking lot is closed), they will have to be either burned for energy or used to build lean body mass.

But suppose we add two slices of whole-wheat toast to the meal. We won't put any butter on the toast; we'll just have it dry. What happens then?

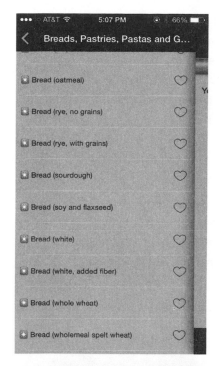

If we go back to the food categories by touching the Add Food button again, and touch the category of Breads, Pastas, Pastries and Grains, we'll get another drop down menu with all the food choices.

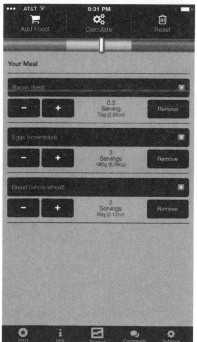

We then add two slices of whole-wheat toast to the meal.

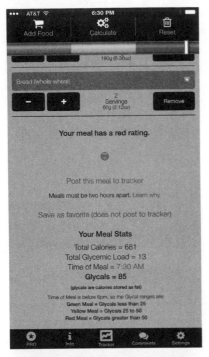

And then we calculate the meal. We can see that we've only added 130 calories to the meal, but the glycemic load has gone from 0 to 13. So, according to what we've learned in Chapter 2, instead of storing 0 percent of the calories as fat, we're now going to store approximately 13 percent of 681 calories (the calories in the meal) as fat, or about 85 calories. This number is a little less than 13 percent because the formula in the app is more complicated than just a straight percentage—but it's a good approximation.

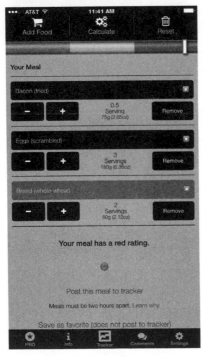

The app will then highlight the worst food in the meal, so you can remove it from the meal by touching the Remove button under the food.

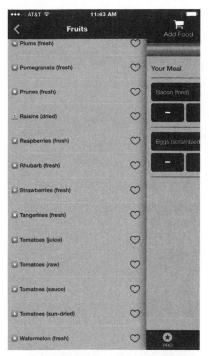

If we remove the whole-wheat toast, we can add another food by touching the Add Food button and going back to the food categories. If we want to substitute strawberries for the whole-wheat toast, we touch the Fruits category and scroll down to strawberries.

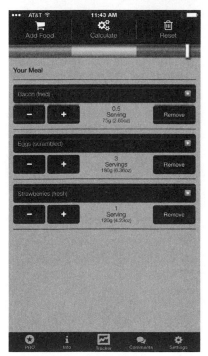

Touching strawberries will add it to the meal in place of the wheat toast.

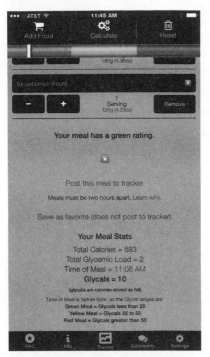

If we then recalculate the meal by touching the Calculate button, we see that the meal has gone from red back to green. Now, the total glycemic load is only 2, so approximately 2 percent of the 583 total calories in the meal—about 10 calories—will be stored as fat.

PORTION SIZE MATTERS!

We've seen how the app accounts for calories and glycemic load, but how *much* you eat at one meal or snack is just as important. For example, if you eat one banana in the morning your meal will look like this:

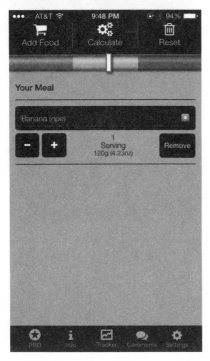

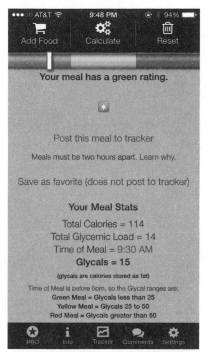

The total number of calories in the banana is 114, the glycemic load (GL) is 14, and the number of glycals (calories stored as fat) is 15. So, this is a green snack.

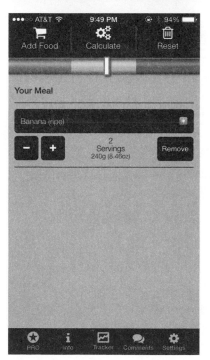

But if you have two bananas at once, your meal will look like this:

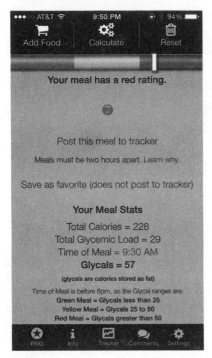

Having two bananas at once doubles the calories, *but it also doubles the glycemic load.* Since the number of glycals depends upon the total calories in the meal *and* the total glycemic load, doubling both will almost *quadruple* the number of glycals.

Eating one banana stores 15 calories as fat; eating two bananas at once stores 57 calories as fat, *almost four times as much!*

HAVE YOUR MAIN MEAL AT LUNCH; EAT LIGHTLY AT NIGHT

When you eat your meal adds another layer of complexity, but the app makes it simple. As we learned in Chapter 2, secreting insulin at night is much worse than earlier in the day because insulin trumps the effects of growth hormone, which peaks at night and is the most important fat-burning hormone in the body. So, an insulin surge in the morning is not as bad as an insulin surge in the evening. That's why people have some successs in losing fat by following the "No carbs after 6 p.m." rule. Restricting carbohydrates at night will lower insulin levels, ensuring the maximum fat-burning affect from the growth hormone you secrete while sleeping. To account for this effect, the app will read the time of day on your phone, and if it's after 6 p.m. the ranges of green, yellow and red become stricter.

The app uses the current time on your phone as the default time of the meal, but you can change the time of the meal by touching the time signature on the results page. Touching the select button recalculates the meal. Changing the time of the meal may change its rating.

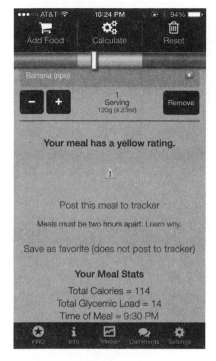

For example, one banana is a green snack in the morning, but a yellow snack at night. Meals must also be two hours apart.

The number of glycals remains unchanged, so you'll store the same amount of fat. But, you'll *burn* less fat by eating the banana at 9:30 p.m. than you would by having it at 9:30 a.m. The change in the rating of the meal warns you that the time of day you have the meal is crucial. In Step 2 of the diet (steady fat loss) you're allowed only one yellow meal a day and one red meal a week, so front-loading your day by eating your main meal (and carbs) earlier in the day will make it easier to follow the diet.

We've seen how the app calculates the amount of fat you store during the day when you're eating, and how the number of calories in the meal, the total glycemic load of the meal, the portion size of the meal and the time between meals affect how much fat you *store*. We've also seen how the time of day of the meal affects how much fat you *burn*. What other factors are important in fat burning?

As you've learned in the previous chapters, when you stop eating at the end of the day and fall asleep, your insulin level drops. This provides a signal to your fat cells to start releasing fat to burn for energy, which is necessary because your body still needs an energy source to continue to function through the night. Insulin levels are lowest when you're sleeping, and the longer you sleep, the more fat you burn.

A high growth hormone level is the second-biggest stimulus to burn fat, and the surge of growth hormone that occurs after you fall asleep is critical in determining how much fat you burn at night. Growth hormone antagonizes the effect of insulin, which is why the amount of fat you have depends on the relative levels of insulin and growth hormone. You know you can minimize insulin levels and fat storage by keeping your meals "green." But how does the app take into account the fat-burning effects of growth hormone?

Growth hormone levels start to decline at about age 20. As growth hormone levels drop, you can actually eat the same diet you have eaten your whole life—maintaining the same insulin levels—but *still* put on fat because as you age there's less opposition to insulin. You have much more leeway with your diet at age 20 than you do at age 50. When you're younger, you can get away with eating junk food occasionally and maintain a trim waistline, but at 50 it's almost impossible. Why? Lower levels of growth hormone. That means you have to be smarter and smarter about your diet as you age if you want to stay slim.

Thyroid hormone levels also decline with age, and levels of thyroid hormone determine how many calories your body burns at rest. People with a low thyroid hormone level will burn fewer calories at night than someone with a higher thyroid hormone level. That's why people with a low-functioning thyroid tend to be overweight; and it's another reason it gets harder to lose fat as you get older.

In my practice, I replace growth hormone and thyroid hormone to more youthful levels, enabling my patients to burn more fat at night and making their fat loss a little easier. But what if you're not replacing the fat-burning hormones? How do you know how many fat calories you're burning at night? How do you figure out the maximum number of calories you can store as fat per day—that is, the maximum number of *glycals* you can have each day—and still lose fat?

There's an app for that, too!

Low Glycal Pro, an in-app paid feature, allows you to enter your personal characteristics, like age, gender, height, weight and average number of hours of sleep per night, to calculate your basal metablolic rate (BMR) and how many fat calories you burn at night. In order to lose fat, you need to store fewer calories during the day than you burn at night. Low Glycal Pro customizes your diet plan by calculating the maximum number of glycals you can have per day and still burn net fat. It also tracks your daily glycals and weight, so you can see at a glance if you're staying in the fat-burning zone, and how it's affecting your weight.

Here's what it looks like:

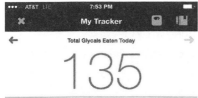

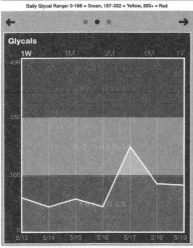

You're also able to store favorite foods and meals, so you can easily access the foods you eat everyday and make small changes to meals without having to enter the entire meal again.

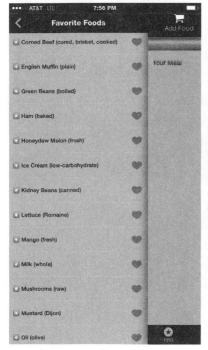

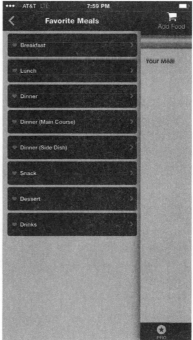

The Low Glycal Diet™ Calculator and Tracker companion app will ensure that you always stay in the "fat-burning zone," whether you're eating at home or on the run. If you make changes to the recipes in this book, you'll be able to see how those changes affect fat storage. You can also check your own recipes easily to make sure they're "green." Often, making small changes, like eliminating the potatoes in your Niçoise salad, or having your toast two hours after your bacon and eggs, will turn your meal from a fat-storing one to a healthy one. The app will tell you when you can eat carbs and when you can't. Your fat loss will be effortless and you'll never be hungry!

You can do this!

CHAPTER 9

DESIGNED FOR SUCCESS: THE TEMPLATE FOR A TRIMMER, YOUNGER YOU— FOR LIFE

Here are three sets of 14-day templates for each step in the 3-step plan of the Low-Glycal Diet. We've said it before (more than once!) but we'll say it again: A written plan will keep you on track with the initial weight loss and with the ongoing long-term maintenance of your ideal weight. When you put pen to paper you are making a commitment that's more powerful than you realize. Plus, we know you'll want to personalize each step of the Low-Glycal Diet to suit your tastes, schedule and budget. Using the templates in this chapter is the easiest way to do that. So take everything you've learned in this book and create a meal plan that works for you.

Start and keep the habit of creating a written meal plan each week. Refer to it as you make your grocery shopping list, and keep a copy of the week's meal plan handy so you can access it easily. This habit will keep you accountable to your diet plan, and happy—grocery shopping will be easier, your food dollars will go farther and you'll be lean and healthy. What's not to like?

I congratulate you on your determination to improve your health and quality of life, and on your pursuit of the Low-Glycal Diet. I created the diet and wrote this book for *you*. Here's to your health. Own it!

MY LOW-GLYCAL DIET MEAL PLAN

Step 1: Kick-Start the Weight Loss

My all low-glycal meal plan for breakfast, lunch, dinner and snacks

WEEK 1	BREAKFAST	SNACK	LUNCH	SNACK	DINNER
MONDAY					
TUESDAY					
WEDNESDAY					
THURSDAY					
FRIDAY					
SATURDAY					
SUNDAY					

Shopping list:

Step 1: Kick-Start the Weight Loss

My all low-glycal meal plan for breakfast, lunch, dinner and snacks

WEEK 2	BREAKFAST	SNACK	LUNCH	SNACK	DINNER
MONDAY					
TUESDAY					
WEDNESDAY					
THURSDAY					
FRIDAY					
SATURDAY					
SUNDAY					

Shopping list:

Step 2: Continue to Lose Weight with a Modified Meal Plan

My low-, medium- and high-glycal meal plan* for breakfast, lunch, dinner and snacks

*All low-glycal except 1 medium-glycal meal a day, and 1 high-glycal meal a week

WEEK 1	BREAKFAST	SNACK	LUNCH	SNACK	DINNER
MONDAY					
TUESDAY					
WEDNESDAY					
THURSDAY					
FRIDAY					
SATURDAY					
SUNDAY					

Shopping list:

Step 2: Continue to Lose Weight with a Modified Meal Plan

My low-, medium- and high-glycal meal plan* for breakfast, lunch, dinner and snacks

*All low-glycal except 1 medium-glycal meal a day, and 1 high-glycal meal a week

WEEK 2	BREAKFAST	SNACK	LUNCH	SNACK	DINNER
MONDAY					
TUESDAY					
WEDNESDAY					
THURSDAY					
FRIDAY					
SATURDAY					
SUNDAY					

Shopping list:

Step 3: Maintain My Ideal Weight

My low-, medium- and high-glycal meal plan* for breakfast, lunch, dinner and snacks

*All low-glycal except 1 medium-glycal meal a day, and 1 high-glycal day a week

WEEK 1	BREAKFAST	SNACK	LUNCH	SNACK	DINNER
MONDAY					
TUESDAY					
WEDNESDAY					
THURSDAY					
FRIDAY					
SATURDAY					
SUNDAY					

Shopping list:

Step 3: Maintain My Ideal Weight

My low-, medium- and high-glycal meal plan* for breakfast, lunch, dinner and snacks

*All low-glycal except 1 medium-glycal meal a day, and 1 high-glycal day a week

WEEK 2	BREAKFAST	SNACK	LUNCH	SNACK	DINNER
MONDAY					
TUESDAY					
WEDNESDAY					
THURSDAY					
FRIDAY					
SATURDAY					
SUNDAY					

Shopping list:

"I'll never go hungry again." – Scarlett O'Hara, *Gone with the Wind*

We all think about food, about treats, about the next meal. We look forward to eating; that's part of being human. When you change your eating habits, and especially with the goal of losing weight, it's important to keep yourself assured that there is food in your future! A written meal plan for the week can be very reassuring when you begin the Low-Glycal Diet. Give yourself a lifeline and make a written meal plan for the week ahead, every week. Whether you are at Step 1 or well into Step 3, you'll be glad to know that you always have something good to eat on the horizon. Ahhh. Take a breath and get back to the rest of your life.

REFERENCES

CHAPTER 1:

Johnston, B., Kanters, S., Bandayrel, K., et al. 2014. "Comparison of Weight Loss Among Named Diet Programs in Overweight and Obese Adults—A Meta-analysis," *JAMA*. September 3; 312(9): 923–933.

American Heart Association (2006). Diet and lifestyle recommendations revision 2006. Circulation, 114(1): 82–96.

Travers, K. 2012. "Six Celebs Who Gained Cash When Losing Weight." In foxbusiness.com/personal-finance/2012/08/09.

Chowdhury, R., Warnakula, S., Kunuysor, S., et al. 2014. "Association of Dietary, Circulating, and Supplement Fatty Acids With Coronary Risk: A Systematic Review and Meta-analysis," *Annals of Internal Medicine*, March 18; 160(6): 398–406.

Atkinson, F., Foster-Powell, K., Brand-Miller, J. 2008. "International Tables of Glycemic Index and Glycemic Load Values: 2008. *Diabetes Care*; 31(12).

CHAPTER 2:

Ebbeling, C., Swain, J., Feldman, H., et al. 2012. "Effects of Dietary Composition on Energy Expenditure During Weight-Loss Maintenance," *JAMA*, June 27: 307(24); 2627–2634.

Proeyen, K., Szlufcik, K., Nielens, H., et al. 2010. "Training in the Fasted State Improves Glucose Tolerance During Fat-Rich Diet," *Journal of Physiology*, November 1; 588(Pt 21): 4289–4302.

Pontzer, H., Raichien, D., Wood, B., et al. 2012. "Hunter-Gatherer Energetics and Human Obesity," *PLoS ONE*, July 25; 7(7): e40503.

Finkel, M. 2009. "The Hazda," *National Geographic Magazine*, December; (12).

Taubes, G. 2008. *Good Calories, Bad Calories*. New York: Anchor Books.

Garaulet, M., Gomez-Abellan, P., Alburquerque-Bejar, J., et al. 2013. "Timing of Food Intake Predicts Weight Loss Effectiveness," *International Journal of Obesity*, April; 37(4): 604–611.

Nedeltcheva, A., Kilkus, J., Imperial, J., et al. 2010. "Insufficient Sleep, Diet, and Obesity," *Annals of Internal Medicine*, October 5; 153(7): 1–28.

Rabbani, N., Godfrey, L., Xue, M., et al. 2011. "Glycation of LDL by Methylglyoxal Increases Arterial Atherogenicity: A Possible Contributor to Increased Risk of Cardiovascular Disease in Diabetes," *Diabetes*, July; 60(7): 1973–1980.

Halton, T., Willett, W., Liu, S., et al. 2006. "Low-Carbohydrate-Diet Score and the Risk of Coronary Heart Disease in Women," *New England Journal of Medicine*, November 9; 355: 1991–2002.

Ho, V., Leung, K., Hsu, A., et al. 2011. "A Low Carbohydrate, High Protein Diet Slows Tumor Growth and Prevents Cancer Initiation," *Cancer Research*, July 1; 71: 4484–4496.

Crane, P., Walker, R., Hubbard, R., et al. 2013. "Glucose Levels and Risk of Dementia," *New England Journal of Medicine*, August 8; 369: 540–548.

Horita, S., Seki, G., Yamada, H., et al. 2011. "Insulin Resistance, Obesity, Hypertension, and Renal Sodium Transport," *International Journal of Hypertension*, Volume 2011 (2011) Article ID 391762, 8 pages.

Whitmer, R., Gustafson, D., Barrett-Conner, E., et al. 2008. "Central Obesity and Increased Risk of Dementia More than Three Decades Later," *Neurology*, September 30; 71(14): 1057–1064.

ACKNOWLEDGMENTS

JEFF: First and foremost, I wish to thank my co-writer, Martha Murphy, without whom this book would not exist. Her talent, experience and encouragement have been invaluable throughout the process of writing this book. A very big thank you to my literary agent, Linda Konner, who believed in this book, helped shape its content and made its publication possible. I'd also like to thank Julie Silver, M.D., at Harvard Medical School, for her continuing education course, "Publishing Books, Memoirs and Other Creative Nonfiction," which gave me the knowledge to navigate the process of publishing a book, and the opportunity to meet some very talented individuals like Martha Murphy and Linda Konner. Thanks to my partner, Mark Henkle, for his encouragement, advice and design of the companion app, and my nephew, Todd Dunham, who wrote the code for the app. Thanks also to Jacques Liberman, a professionally trained French chef, who contributed some of the recipes for the book. And lastly, I'd like to thank my patients, for their trust in me and inspiration over the last 12 years. They've shown me what works and what doesn't, and have given me the clinical experience necessary to hone and refine the Low-Glycal Diet into what it is today.

MARTHA: My thanks to Julie Silver, MD, for inviting me to teach at her annual CME conference, where I met Jeff Dunham and learned about the glycal. Thank you, Jeff, for choosing me to work with you on your book—it's been an honor. Thanks also to Linda Konner, literary agent, for championing the proposal; to Will Kiester at Page Street Publishing for his enthusiasm for this project; and to Linda Beaulieu—a life-saver when I was down to the wire writing recipes. I am eternally grateful for the good fortune I had to be born into a family of thoughtful, inquisitive people. As always: thank you, Kevin, for being there.

ABOUT THE AUTHORS

Jeffrey S. Dunham, M.D., Ph.D., M.P.H.

Jeffrey S. Dunham, M.D., Ph.D., M.P.H. is Medical Director of BioFit Medical Group in Palm Springs, California, and specializes in Anti-Aging and Preventive Medicine. He has an M.D. from Harvard Medical School, a Ph.D. in Biology from M.I.T., and a M.P.H. from the University of California, Berkeley. He is certified by the American Board of Preventive Medicine and is a member of the American Academy of Anti-Aging Medicine.

Martha W. Murphy

Martha Murphy is an award-winning writer with an interest in health, healthcare and medicine; food and the people who bring it to us; entrepreneurs; and life in out-of-the-way places.

INDEX